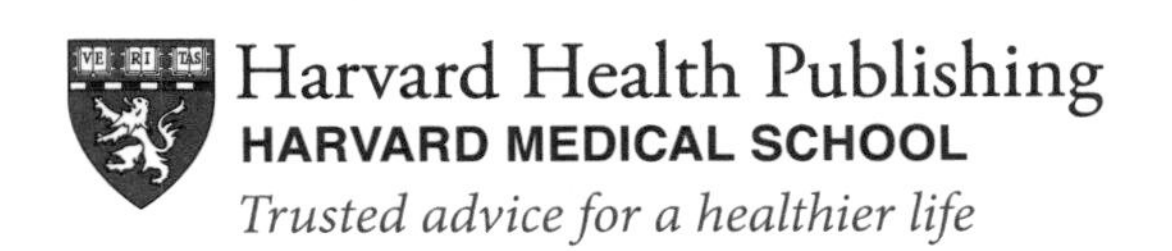

Dear Reader,

Out of sight, out of mind, your digestive system is working around the clock delivering the nutrients in food to your bloodstream. As long as the system is running smoothly, you need not think about it. Once trouble begins, however, your gut—like a squeaky wheel—suddenly demands your attention.

For some folks, symptoms such as diarrhea, gas, cramps, heartburn, indigestion, nausea, belching, bloating, and constipation are infrequent and tolerable, but many people experience them far more often. An estimated one in four people has frequent gastrointestinal problems that can severely disrupt a normal lifestyle. And the number of prescriptions for gastrointestinal medications has soared since the late 1990s, according to federal statistics.

Although these symptoms—and the misery they inflict—are real, they often can't be attributed to a detectable physical cause, such as a structural abnormality, hormonal change, or infection. In such a case, doctors call the problem a functional disorder (as opposed to an organic one, which has an identifiable cause). Functional cases make up about 40% of all diagnoses made by gastroenterologists. Physicians and scientists take these disorders seriously and, as research continues, it is likely that subtle changes will be found to be responsible for more of them, taking them out of the realm of functional disorders.

This report focuses on a number of disorders that are often considered to be functional—reflux, dyspepsia, irritable bowel syndrome, constipation, diarrhea, excessive gas, and belly pain—although most of these also have identifiable causes in some cases. If your symptoms occur frequently, last more than a month or two, or interfere greatly with normal activities, it's a good idea to seek help. Even when doctors can't pinpoint an underlying physical cause for your symptoms, they can still provide insight into what's happening in your gut and offer strategies for gaining relief.

The good news is that our ability to treat gastrointestinal disorders (functional and otherwise) continues to improve. With proper knowledge—and the support of the right combination of health professionals—you can make changes in your lifestyle, use specific medications, find other helpful therapies that will ease your discomfort, and make the right decisions about medical treatments.

Sincerely,

Lawrence S. Friedman, MD

Lawrence S. Friedman, M.D.
Medical Editor

Harvard Health Publishing | Harvard Medical School | 4 Blackfan Circle, 4th Floor | Boston, MA 02115

Inside the gut

The "gut." It's an ancient Anglo-Saxon word that refers to the human digestive system. Think of this superb accomplishment of nature's engineering as a perpetual food processor, constantly mixing, grinding, and transforming the meats, vegetables, fruits, and snacks that you eat into biologically useful molecules.

Nearly 30 feet long if stretched out straight, the gut is a series of hollow organs linked to form a long, twisting tube that runs from the mouth to the anus (see Figure 1, at right). This string of organs is known variously as the alimentary canal, gastrointestinal tract, or digestive tract. It comprises the esophagus (or gullet), stomach, small intestine, and colon (which includes the rectum). These organs break down food and liquids—carbohydrates, fats, and proteins—into chemical components that the body can absorb as nutrients and use for energy or to build or repair cells. What's left is expelled by a highly efficient disposal system.

The organs of the gut are almost always moving, driven by muscles in their walls. These muscles consist of an outer longitudinal layer and an inner circular layer. The coordinated contractions of these layers push food and fluids the length of the canal. If you've ever seen a video of a snake swallowing a mouse, you've got some idea of what the process is like. This dynamic movement along the gastrointestinal tract is known as peristalsis.

Helping with the job of digestion is the mucosa, or lining, of the mouth, stomach, and small intestine, which harbors glands that produce digestive enzymes. The salivary glands, liver, and pancreas also secrete juices that help make food soluble (dissolvable in water) so that nutrients can pass easily into the bloodstream.

The digestive journey

Pop a grape, chocolate, or shrimp into your mouth. Immediately, digestion begins. In the mouth itself, the tongue and teeth help to get the process started by chewing and chopping the food so it's small enough to swallow. Salivary glands secrete saliva, releasing an enzyme that changes some starches into simple sugars and softens the food for swallowing. The saliva also allows the taste buds of the tongue to sense the flavors of your foods.

Swallowing is a complicated, coordinated act that begins when your tongue pushes food back into your throat, or pharynx. This voluntary action sets off an involuntary chain of events that transports the food from the throat into the esophagus and down

Figure 1: A lengthy journey

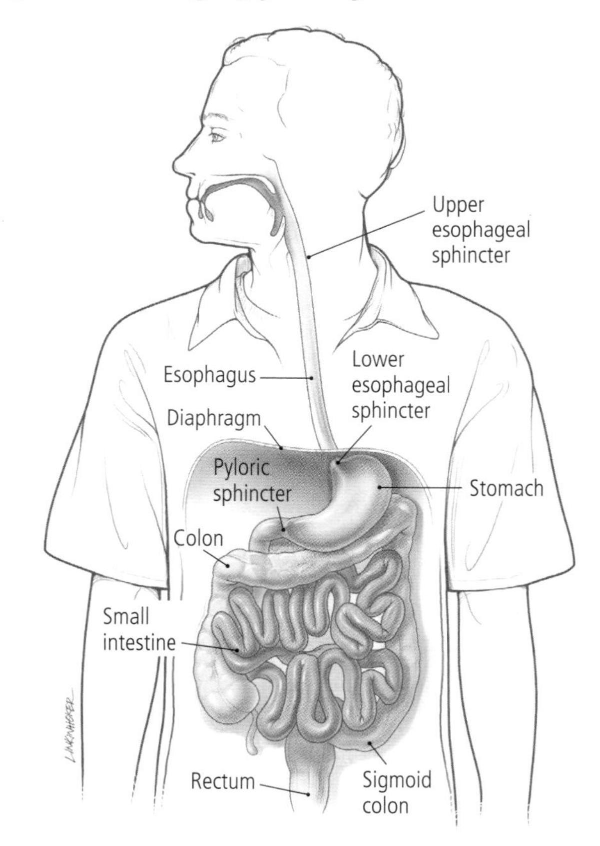

The food you eat travels a winding 30-foot pathway known as the gastrointestinal tract or the alimentary canal. Along the way, the mucosa—the surface layer of cells lining the gastrointestinal tract—produces digestive enzymes and juices that help break down food to be absorbed into the bloodstream.

into the stomach, a journey that typically takes eight seconds (see Figure 2, at right).

Esophagus

Food does not simply drop down the esophagus by means of gravity. Matter moves through this passageway because it is pushed by contractions of the esophageal muscles.

Think of the esophagus (along with the intestine) as an empty tube surrounded by layers of muscle that contract in a succession of waves. As the ball of food, called a bolus, travels toward the far end of the 10- to 13-inch-long tube, the lower esophageal sphincter—one of several cylindrical muscles along the digestive tract that function as gates—opens to allow the food to enter the stomach, then closes again. The esophageal tube is quite elastic, stretching to nearly two inches across to accommodate foods of various sizes.

While the esophagus is moving things along, it also has to keep food from backing up (regurgitating) and re-entering the throat. That's where a muscle known as the upper esophageal sphincter comes into play. The two esophageal sphincters, upper and lower, make sure the food doesn't travel in the wrong direction.

Stomach

If the esophagus is a conduit with a valve at each end, the stomach is like a storage and processing facility, where the food is prepared for digestion.

This food warehouse can accommodate anything from a light afternoon snack to a five-course meal.

Figure 2: How long does it take?

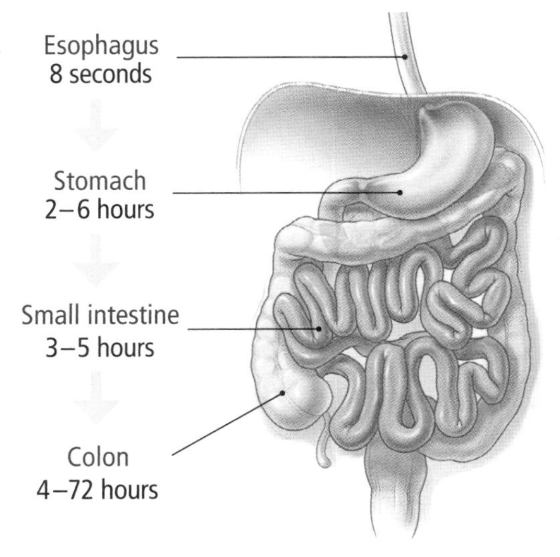

The time it takes for food to pass all the way through the digestive tract can be anywhere from nine hours to over three days depending on the content of the meal and your body's unique physiology.

Without this large storage capacity, you'd have to eat small, frequent meals, and you'd be unable to drink large quantities of liquids at any given time.

But the stomach doesn't just hold food: muscles in the lower stomach (see Figure 3, below) also mix that food into a soft mush. This process is aided by the liquids you drink and by saliva, hydrochloric acid, and the enzyme pepsin. Hydrochloric acid and pepsin, produced by the glands that line the stomach, help break down proteins into their constituent amino acids. The stomach mucosa has a defense system, including an overlying layer of mucus and bicar-

Figure 3: The stomach wall

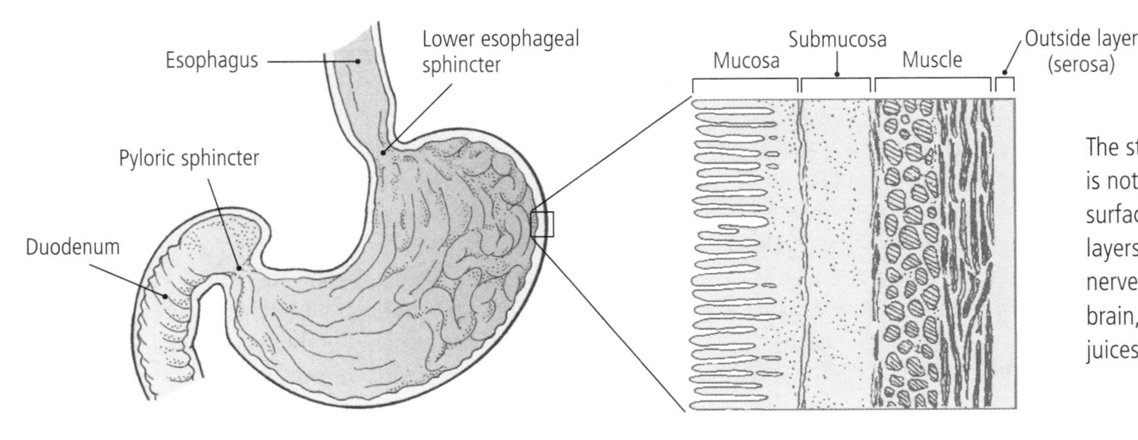

The stomach lining (mucosa) is not a smooth, balloon-like surface. Instead, it has several layers that contain muscles, nerve connections to the brain, and glands that secrete juices to help digest food.

bonate, to protect itself. After mixing, a once-palatable meal is reduced to a thick liquid called chyme.

The other important function of the stomach is delivering the resulting chyme to the small intestine in amounts it can handle. The involuntary contractions that push stomach contents along are governed by nerves in the stomach wall, which transmit electrical impulses to the brain. The nerves that carry impulses from the gastrointestinal tract, called visceral nerves, recognize stretching, pulling, or expansion (distension) of the muscles in the walls of the digestive tract. Pain can result when these sensations are excessive.

When you haven't eaten for a while and your stomach is empty, it initiates a series of rhythmic contractions known as hunger pangs. They serve as a signal to the brain: "Feed me!" These contractions explain stomach noises, which also can occur when air or fluid is moving around inside. Once you've eaten, it takes about two hours for the muscular stomach to reduce a typical meal to a liquid and have it ready to move along to the small intestine. A high-protein meal can take an extra hour or two. A high-fat meal can take up to six hours. That's why foods with healthy fats (such as those in nuts) help you feel full longer than high-carbohydrate foods like sugary snacks.

Small intestine

Through another gate called the pyloric sphincter, the stomach empties the chyme into the small intestine. This hollow tube, which is a remarkable 21 feet long, is where the main work of digestion takes place. The small intestine breaks down fats, starches, and proteins into fatty acids, simple sugars, and amino acids, which it can then absorb.

A living colony in your gut—that's a good thing

The digestive tract is filled with living microorganisms, collectively called the microbiota or microbiome. A healthy and varied bacterial ecosystem is important for proper gastrointestinal function and for maintaining robust health in general.

That said, individuals vary greatly in their microbiomes. The basics are set early in life and are influenced by a variety of factors, including whether or not you were breastfed or delivered vaginally, whether your mother took any antibiotics during pregnancy for an infection, and even early life events, such as trauma. Throughout your life, your diet is an important factor that can alter the composition of the microbiome in your gut (see "Probiotics and prebiotics," page 28). And at any age, any antibiotics you take to kill off disease-causing bacteria somewhere in your body also kill off bacteria in the gut, which can throw the microbiome out of balance. In general, older people have fewer species of bacteria in the digestive tract, perhaps as an effect of aging itself or the accumulated impact of dietary changes and the use of antibiotics and other medications.

That's important because the microorganisms in your gut produce about half a million different molecules, and these substances communicate with your brain as well as the nerves, immune system, and endocrine cells in your gastrointestinal tract. As one example, production of the neurotransmitter serotonin—which plays a role in mood, sleep, and pain sensitivity—occurs mainly in the gut, spurred by signals from the microbiome. Through the action of the microbiome, your diet influences how much serotonin you produce. The microbiome has also been linked to obesity, inflammation, and even Parkinson's disease.

While many of the bacteria in your gut carry out essential, health-promoting tasks, others can cause problems, such as diarrhea or dysentery. Under normal circumstances, the "good" bacteria keep the "bad" bacteria in check. However, some of the conditions described in this report appear to involve an excess of "bad" bacteria. For example, a less diverse microbiome may increase constipation. It can also lower the body's defense against gastrointestinal infections and increase inflammation in the gut.

When it comes to irritable bowel syndrome (IBS) or other functional gastrointestinal disorders, there isn't a specific pattern of microorganisms to point to, but there's lots of indirect evidence that your gut bacteria are involved. For example, a major assault on your gastrointestinal microbiome, such as viral gastroenteritis (a gut infection), sometimes induces IBS. Infection of the stomach with the *Helicobacter pylori* bacterium can cause dyspepsia. An excess (overgrowth) of bacteria in the small intestine can also cause IBS symptoms, which in this case can be eased by treatment with certain antibiotics. In some people, IBS symptoms are related to substances produced when bacteria in the intestine digest certain carbohydrates, and eliminating these foods from the diet reduces symptoms. There are even attempts to directly alter the microbiome in people with IBS by using fecal transplants from healthy people, but this is by no means standard therapy (see "A new treatment for IBS?" on page 28).

The food you eat generally takes three to five hours to move through the small intestine. During this time, the food is bathed in digestive enzymes and juices that flow into the intestine through ducts from the liver and pancreas. Bile, produced by the liver and stored in the gallbladder, emulsifies fat, enabling its absorption. Enzymes secreted by the pancreas, such as trypsin, amylase, and lipase, help digest proteins, carbohydrates, and fats. Once reduced to products the body can manage, the nutrients from digested food are absorbed by the intestine's thin lining and sent to cells throughout the body by way of the bloodstream and lymphatic system.

The small intestine is divided into three parts, and each serves a somewhat different digestive function.

- First is the foot-long duodenum, located a few inches above the navel. Many minerals, such as iron and calcium, are absorbed into the body through the duodenum. This is also where bile and pancreatic juices join the mix.
- After the duodenum, the next part of the small intestine is the jejunum, which measures eight feet in length. In the jejunum, fats, starches, and proteins are further broken down and absorbed.
- The third and lowest portion of the small intestine, the ileum, is approximately 12 feet long. The ileum absorbs water, as well as vitamin B_{12} and bile salts.

Colon (large intestine)

Finally, what's left of the food arrives in the colon, or large intestine, a four-foot-long muscular tube about the diameter of your fist, where the walls act like a sponge and soak up 80% to 90% of the remaining water. In fact, the colon accepts about a quart of liquid from the ileum each day. Once inside the colon, food residue travels up the right side (the ascending colon), across the body (in the transverse colon), down the left side (the descending colon), through the sigmoid colon to the rectum, and out of the body. The time required for food to move through the colon varies widely, but is generally in the range of four to 72 hours.

Bacteria that reside in the colon help in the digestive process, feeding off whatever remains of your meal. The bacteria produce fatty acids as well as hydrogen, carbon dioxide, and, in some people, methane gas. Some of these gases are consumed as nutrients by the cells of the colon, while others are expelled as waste. Undigested matter, such as fiber, is propelled along by contractions of the colon wall and settles as solids in the rectum, the final six inches of the colon.

The end of the rectum is guarded by a pair of sphincter muscles that help control what goes out. The waste accumulates until the rectal wall becomes so distended that it signals the internal anal sphincter to relax, triggering the urge for a bowel movement. The external anal sphincter, which is under voluntary control, keeps the rectal contents in place until a convenient time.

What comes out is primarily water and colon bacteria (see "A living colony in your gut—that's a good thing," page 4), plus bile, mucus, and cells normally shed from the intestinal lining. Undigested food makes up very little of the average quarter- to half-pound stool. The exception is fiber: the more fiber you ingest, the greater the quantity of your stool.

Gastroesophageal reflux disease

Heartburn, that uncomfortable burning sensation that radiates up the middle of your chest, is the most common gastrointestinal complaint. Heartburn is often an indicator of a condition known as gastroesophageal reflux disease (GERD, or just "reflux"), in which acid, pepsin, or both rise from the stomach into the esophagus, much like water bubbling into a sink from a plugged drain.

Episodes of reflux often go unnoticed, but when reflux is excessive and frequent, the gastric juices irritate the esophagus, producing the pain of heartburn. The burning sensation is usually felt in the chest just behind the breastbone and often extends from the lower end of the rib cage to the root of the neck. It can last for hours and is sometimes accompanied by the very unpleasant, stinging, sour sensation of highly acidic fluid rushing into the back of the throat. Sometimes acid regurgitates all the way up to the mouth and may come up forcefully as vomit or as a "wet burp." It can hit as you sit in a traffic jam, after you eat spicy foods, or when you lie down in bed. Many women experience this sensation during pregnancy. Heartburn can be so intense that you think you are having a heart attack. Although heartburn can be extremely painful, it is not generally a serious threat to your health.

More people are suffering with this and other symptoms of GERD than ever before. In one survey, 59% of participants said they had experienced heartburn in the previous week, and more than one-third said they had experienced reflux. This epidemic leads people to spend $2.6 billion a year on over-the-counter heartburn remedies. Clearly, it's a major problem.

Help is available, however. GERD can be aggravated by many things, ranging from emotional stress to a variety of foods and even particular body positions, like reclining or bending forward. Many people manage quite well by controlling such things as stress, diet, or position. There are also medications and surgical options available.

Figure 4: Reflux

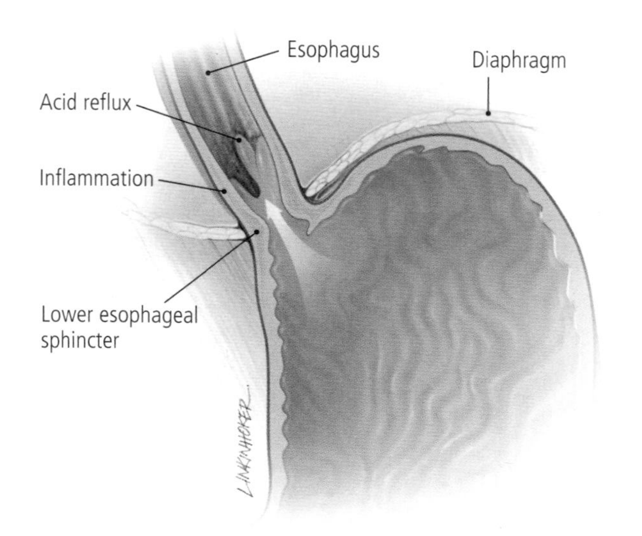

Gastroesophageal reflux disease is an often-painful condition that occurs when the lower esophageal sphincter fails to do its job of keeping digestive juices in the stomach. When the sphincter relaxes too much, acidic stomach fluids surge up into the esophagus, sometimes causing a painful burning sensation behind the breastbone known as heartburn. In some cases, this also causes inflammation in the lining of the esophagus.

Causes of reflux

GERD is a digestive disorder affecting the lower esophageal sphincter (LES), the muscle connecting the esophagus and stomach. This muscle acts as a barrier to protect the esophagus against the backflow of gastric acid from the stomach. Normally, it works something like a gate, opening to allow food to pass into the stomach and closing to keep food and acidic stomach juices from flowing back into the esophagus.

The LES is a complex segment of smooth muscle under the control of nerves and various hormones. As a result, dietary substances, drugs, and nervous system factors can impair its function. Gastroesophageal reflux occurs when the LES weakens or just relaxes when it shouldn't, allowing contents of the stomach to rise up into the esophagus (see Figure 4, page 6). Scientists aren't always sure exactly why this happens, but they have identified some contributing factors.

Digestive abnormalities. Malfunction of the LES isn't the only digestive problem that can contribute to reflux and heartburn. If stomach muscles don't contract normally, this can delay the emptying of the stomach, increasing the risk that acid will reflux back into the esophagus. In addition, esophageal contractions that should clear refluxed acid may fail to do so. There could also be a reduction in the esophageal lining's ability to resist damage, or a decrease in production of saliva (which has a neutralizing effect on acid).

Weight. Being overweight increases the risk of frequent GERD symptoms. Even if a person's body mass index (BMI, a ratio of weight to height) remains in the normal range, weight gain may bring on heartburn. The additional weight can increase pressure on the stomach, pushing its contents up.

Pregnancy. Pregnancy can promote GERD, both because of hormonal changes and because the enlarging uterus presses against other organs.

Age. As you age, esophageal contractions and the muscles of the LES may weaken. However, since the esophagus can become less sensitive to acid with age, reflux might not result in heartburn. Instead, you may feel nausea or vague chest discomfort.

Foods and drinks. Diet can contribute to dysfunction of the LES. For example, alcohol can loosen the LES (and irritate the esophageal lining), as can coffee and other caffeine-containing products. Coffee, tea, cocoa, and cola drinks are all powerful stimulants of gastric acid production. Mints and chocolate, often served to cap off a meal to aid in digestion, can relax the LES and can induce heartburn. Some people say that onions and garlic give them heartburn. Others have trouble with citrus fruits or tomato products, which can irritate the esophageal lining. High-fat and fried foods can also trigger symptoms. If you notice that a particular food leads to episodes of heartburn, by all means, stay away from it.

Eating patterns. How you eat can be as important as what you eat. Skipping some meals and then eating heavily can increase pressure in the stomach and the possibility of reflux. Lying down right after eating will only make the problem worse. It is best to wait three hours after eating before going to bed. And stay away from late-night snacks.

Medications. Some prescription drugs can worsen your heartburn (see Table 1, below). Oral contraceptives or postmenopausal hormone preparations containing progesterone are known culprits. Aspirin and other nonsteroidal anti-inflammatory drugs

Table 1: Common medications that can cause reflux

This table shows examples of each class; not all brands or versions are listed.

GENERIC NAME	BRAND NAME(S)	USE
Bronchodilators		
theophylline	Aerolate, Uniphyl, others	Relieves wheezing
Calcium-channel blockers		
amlodipine	Norvasc	Lower blood pressure and improve coronary artery blood flow
diltiazem	Cardizem	
nifedipine	Adalat, Procardia	
verapamil	Calan, Isoptin	
Nonsteroidal anti-inflammatory drugs (NSAIDs)		
aspirin	Bufferin, Ecotrin, others	Relieve pain and inflammation
ibuprofen	Advil, Motrin	
naproxen	Aleve, Anaprox, Naprosyn	
Osteoporosis drugs		
alendronate	Fosamax	Build bone density
ibandronate	Boniva	
risedronate	Actonel	
Progestins		
medroxy-progesterone acetate	Depo-Provera, Provera	Relieve symptoms of menopause; used in oral contraceptives
norethindrone acetate	Aygestin, Micronor	
Tricyclic antidepressants		
amitriptyline	Elavil, Endep	Relieve depression; occasionally used for long-term pain
nortriptyline	Aventyl, Pamelor	
protriptyline	Vivactil	

(NSAIDs) such as ibuprofen (Advil, Motrin) and naproxen (Aleve, Naprosyn) may also pose problems. Corticosteroids are also known to cause heartburn. Osteoporosis drugs such as alendronate (Fosamax) irritate the esophagus. And some antidepressants, tranquilizers, and calcium-channel blockers (used to treat high blood pressure or coronary artery disease) can contribute to reflux by relaxing the LES. The asthma medication theophylline may initiate or aggravate reflux in some people.

To prevent medications from irritating your esophagus, take a few sips of water before you swallow a pill and drink a cup of liquid afterward to speed the pill's transit through your esophagus into your stomach. If you take any drugs known to irritate the esophagus, such as alendronate, stand or sit upright for at least 30 minutes after taking the pill.

Smoking. Smoking can irritate the entire digestive tract and may also relax the LES. In addition, frequent sucking on a cigarette can cause you to swallow air, increasing stomach pressure and encouraging reflux.

Hiatal hernia. Hiatal hernia is a common condition that develops when part of the stomach pushes up through the diaphragm—the band of muscle that separates the chest from the abdomen and helps with breathing. The diaphragm has a small opening (hiatus), which should be just large enough for the esophagus to pass through. However, in a person with hiatal hernia, part of the stomach also protrudes through the diaphragm and into the chest (see Figure 5, above right). This impairs the LES's ability to prevent reflux, particularly if the hiatal hernia is large.

Other medical conditions. As many as 70% of people with asthma have reflux. It's not clear, however, whether asthma is a cause or an effect. Still, asthma often improves when GERD is treated. Other illnesses that sometimes contribute to reflux include diabetes, ulcers, and some types of cancer.

Figure 5: Hiatal hernia

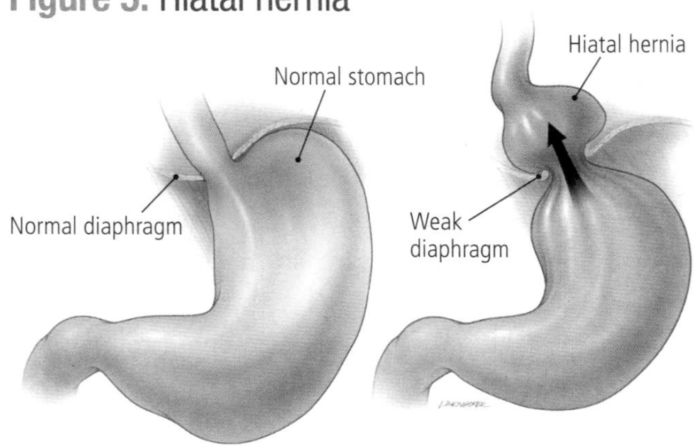

One factor that may contribute to heartburn is a common condition called hiatal hernia, in which a portion of the stomach protrudes through the opening in a weak diaphragm, the band of muscle that separates the chest from the abdomen.

Diagnosing reflux

Many people can manage heartburn through dietary changes and over-the-counter medications (see "Self-help for reflux," page 10). A doctor can be helpful if your symptoms don't respond to self-help techniques and they interfere with sleep or daily life. If you do seek your physician's advice, a detailed account of your symptoms (including when they occur in relation to when you eat and specific foods you consume) will help him or her make the diagnosis.

The doctor will review your medical history and ask questions about the nature of the pain and its pattern of onset. For example, he or she might ask whether symptoms are worse after you eat a heavy meal or known dietary troublemakers such as high-fat foods. Your doctor will want to know if bending over to tie your shoelaces or lying down aggravates the symptoms, and whether the pain seems linked to anxiety or stress.

For typical reflux symptoms, doctors usually forgo diagnostic tests and proceed straight to treatment, starting with a proton-pump inhibitor (PPI) such as omeprazole (Prilosec, Zegerid) or lansoprazole (Prevacid). If these acid-suppressing medications provide relief, the odds are that the diagnosis of GERD was correct. Once symptoms are under control, you may either continue with the PPI or switch to a less powerful medication. That might be a histamine$_2$-receptor antagonist (H2 blocker) such as cimetidine (Tagamet), ranitidine (Zantac), or famotidine (Pepcid), or an antacid like Tums. If the medicine doesn't relieve your symptoms or if other symptoms need investigation, the doctor might order diagnostic tests to detect reflux or inflammation in the esophagus, measure pH levels in the esophagus, or rule out other conditions (see "Do you need diagnostic testing?" below).

Your doctor will be alert for other symptoms, such as frequent nonburning chest pain, bleeding into the gastrointestinal tract, dysphagia (difficulty in swallowing), hoarseness, or constant coughing and wheezing. Such symptoms may be associated with GERD but could have other causes and might warrant tests to gain more information.

For example, GERD is sometimes accompanied by respiratory or throat problems such as asthmatic wheezing, coughing, or hoarseness. When asthma strikes adult nonsmokers with no history of lung disease or allergies, pH-monitoring studies sometimes suggest that GERD is the culprit.

Experts now divide heartburn into four categories, depending on symptoms and test results:

- **Erosive esophagitis.** The lining of the esophagus is already inflamed and worn away in spots as a result of acid exposure (see "Esophagitis," page 10).
- **Non-erosive reflux disease.** There is an abnormal amount of acid reflux but no inflammation seen in the lining of the esophagus.
- **Reflux hypersensitivity.** Acid induces heartburn symptoms, but the amount of acid that is refluxed is normal.
- **Functional heartburn.** Heartburn occurs despite an absence of reflux or excessive sensitivity to acid (see "Do you have functional heartburn?" on page 10).

Identifying the correct category in an individual patient helps ensure appropriate treatment.

Complications of reflux

Although simple reflux is uncomfortable, it doesn't usually pose a danger to healthy individuals. Half to three-quarters of people with reflux disease have mild symptoms that generally clear up in response to simple

Do you need diagnostic testing?

Doctors ordinarily don't put people with heartburn through costly diagnostic evaluations. However, more serious reflux symptoms—such as bleeding from the esophagus, swallowing problems, or severe symptoms that fail to respond to standard treatment for GERD—might warrant further investigation. People who haven't found relief with medications might also benefit from testing, usually performed while they are not taking the drugs. Common tests include the following:

Upper GI endoscopy. This is a method of viewing the inside of the esophagus to look for signs of inflammation or tissue damage. Upper GI endoscopy (the GI is short for gastrointestinal) is considered the gold standard for testing for GERD. For this test, the physician uses a flexible tube that's about as wide as a finger. After giving the person a sedative and depressing the gag reflex with a local anesthetic spray, the doctor passes the tube through the person's mouth and down the throat. The tube contains a light and camera, which allow the doctor to inspect the lining of the esophagus, assess injuries such as ulcers or strictures, and take a biopsy (a tissue sample), if necessary.

Transnasal esophagoscopy. This technique, which is available only in some facilities, uses a scope that is smaller than a standard endoscope; it is about the size of a straw. The physician inserts the scope through the nose down to the esophagus. No sedation is needed, it can be done in the doctor's office, and people can see the images and learn the results immediately. This test is not yet widely used, but it may gain popularity in the future for screening people with GERD for Barrett's esophagus (a change in the lining of the esophagus that occasionally predisposes to esophageal cancer).

Monitoring pH. These tests monitor an individual's reflux episodes over a day or two and measure pH (acidity) levels in the esophagus. One method involves using endoscopy to insert a small capsule in the esophagus. The capsule is clipped in place for 48 hours, while a radio transmitter records pH levels. People can keep track of the times when they eat or sleep and find out how their pH levels correlate with these activities. The doctor might ask the person to stop taking medication during this time to see how the pH level responds without medication.

In another method, the doctor passes a thin, acid-sensing probe through the nose and positions it just above the LES. The probe stays in place for 24 hours to assess pH and reflux levels.

Impedance testing. This is a more sophisticated testing method requiring specialized training. Impedance testing monitors both acid and non-acid reflux. The doctor passes a flexible catheter through the nose and down into the esophagus. Sensors at the end of the catheter relay information to a recording device. You wear the impedance device overnight while going about your normal activity. It is particularly useful for people who have non-acid reflux (when low-acid stomach contents rise into the esophagus).

measures. Over time, however, serious problems can develop when GERD goes untreated or when treatment is ineffective. These complications can include narrowing (stricture) of the esophagus, erosion of its lining, precancerous changes in its cells, and esophageal ulcers.

Esophagitis. One complication, known as reflux esophagitis or erosive esophagitis, is inflammation that occurs when acid and pepsin, released from the stomach, erode areas of the mucosa, the surface layer of cells that line the esophagus. Besides the burning sensation of heartburn, people with esophagitis may also feel pain spreading into the back or up to the neck, jaw, or even the ears. Occasionally, the pain can be so intense that you have trouble swallowing, and you may even think you are having a heart attack.

With esophagitis, food may feel as if it sticks in your throat before going down. Hot drinks may be unpleasant to swallow, and you might have some nausea. You might also regurgitate some acidic fluid into your throat, resulting in a cough. The inflammation of the esophagus can even lead to bleeding. Upper GI endoscopy (see "Do you need diagnostic testing?" on page 9) can confirm the diagnosis of esophagitis and locate any associated ulcers or strictures. Bleeding ulcers in an inflamed esophagus may require aggressive treatment, such as blood transfusions and a procedure to stop the bleeding. To do this, the doctor will pass a probe into the throat through an endoscopic tube and seal off the bleeding area by applying electricity or heat, injecting a substance that constricts blood vessels, or placing a tiny clip on a bleeding vessel.

Barrett's esophagus. Another complication of chronic esophageal inflammation is Barrett's esophagus, an abnormality in which tall cells resembling those that line the small intestine replace the flat squamous cells that normally line the lower esophagus. The condition, a potential consequence of longstanding GERD, is caused by long-term and severe exposure to stomach acid and, in some cases, bile from the small intestine that has refluxed through the stomach and into the esophagus. White men over age 50 who developed GERD at an early age and have had it for many years are at the highest risk for getting Barrett's esophagus and are most likely to be advised to undergo an endoscopy to look for signs of it.

Do you have functional heartburn?

Functional heartburn is heartburn whose symptoms cannot be linked to acid reflux or a structural abnormality. To be diagnosed with functional heartburn, you must have experienced all of the following for the past three months, with symptoms starting at least six months before diagnosis:

- ✔ burning discomfort or pain behind the breastbone
- ✔ no evidence that symptoms are caused by excessive acid refluxed from the stomach into the esophagus or by increased sensitivity of the lining of the esophagus to acid
- ✔ lack of relief from drugs that decrease acid secretion
- ✔ absence of structural disorders that interfere with the movement of food down the esophagus.

These criteria come from a group of more than 100 international experts and are known as the Rome criteria. They cover all functional gastrointestinal disorders, including functional heartburn. As this report went to press, the most recent version available was Rome IV, published in 2016.

Barrett's esophagus can, over time, develop into cancer, but the risk appears to be very small—between one-tenth and one-half of 1%, depending on whether abnormal cells were detected when the endoscopy was performed to make the Barrett's diagnosis. Currently, people with Barrett's esophagus are typically advised to have regular endoscopic evaluations with biopsies (called surveillance endoscopies) to identify abnormal cells. Consult your physician about your initial test results and how often you should be checked for esophageal cancer.

Other problems. GERD can also result in dental problems, including loss of tooth enamel. And it can cause spasms of the vocal cords (larynx), blocking the flow of air to the lungs. One study has reported that such spasms can cause sleep apnea, a condition in which breathing repeatedly stops and starts during sleep.

Self-help for reflux

Modifying diet and lifestyle remains the foundation for treating the symptoms of reflux. Doctors particularly recommend lifestyle changes for people with mild GERD symptoms or symptoms that are not relieved by acid-reducing medications. The following strategies help you prevent heartburn and other symptoms by avoiding foods that reduce the effectiveness of the LES and keeping stomach contents where they belong.

Eat smaller meals. A large meal remains in the stomach for several hours, increasing the chances for gastroesophageal reflux. Try distributing your daily food intake over three, four, or five smaller meals.

Relax when you eat. Stress increases the production of stomach acid, so make meals a pleasant, relaxing experience. Sit down. Eat slowly. Chew completely. Play soothing music.

Relax between meals. Relaxation therapies such as deep breathing, meditation, massage, tai chi, or yoga may help prevent and relieve heartburn. (See the Special Section, "The stress connection," page 30.)

Remain upright after eating. You should maintain postures that reduce the risk for reflux for at least three hours after eating. For example, don't bend over or strain to lift heavy objects.

Avoid eating within three hours of going to bed. Lying down after eating will increase chances of reflux.

Lose weight. Excess pounds increase pressure on the stomach and can push acid into the esophagus.

Loosen up. Avoid tight belts, waistbands, and other clothing that puts pressure on your stomach.

Avoid foods that burn. Abstain from food or drink that increases gastric acid secretion, decreases LES pressure, or slows the emptying of the stomach. Known offenders include high-fat foods, spicy dishes, tomatoes and tomato products, citrus fruits, garlic, onions, milk, carbonated drinks, coffee (including decaf), tea, chocolate, mints, and alcohol. The list is long, but you're likely to see a substantial improvement if you cut out or minimize such foods.

Stop smoking. Nicotine stimulates stomach acid and impairs LES function.

Chew gum. It can increase saliva production, soothing the esophagus and neutralizing acid and washing it back down to the stomach.

Consult your doctor about your medications. Drugs that can predispose you to reflux include aspirin and other NSAIDs, oral contraceptives, hormone therapy drugs, certain antidepressants, and some asthma medications (see Table 1, page 7).

Sleep at an angle. If you're bothered by nighttime heartburn, place a wedge (available in medical supply stores) under your upper body. But don't elevate your head with extra pillows. That makes reflux worse by bending you at the waist and compressing your stomach. You might also try sleeping on your left side, as studies have shown this to reduce reflux—perhaps because the stomach is on the left side of the body, so lying on your left positions most of the stomach below the level of the LES.

Exercise wisely. Wait at least two hours after a meal before engaging in vigorous activity, giving your stomach time to empty.

What else could it be?

Heartburn can be a symptom of GERD, but it can also be a symptom of a condition called eosinophilic esophagitis. This is a disease characterized by the presence of eosinophils (a type of white blood cell associated with allergic reactions) in the wall of the esophagus, where they stimulate inflammation. In addition to heartburn, eosinophilic esophagitis can cause dysphagia, the feeling of food or pills sticking in your esophagus. The disease often occurs in children and young adults, many of whom also have allergies or asthma.

If your symptoms and the appearance of the esophagus on endoscopy (see "Do you need diagnostic testing?" on page 9) seem to indicate eosinophilic esophagitis, a proton-pump inhibitor such as omeprazole (Prilosec) or lansoprazole (Prevacid) is usually the first recommendation. If that doesn't work, your doctor may suggest that you eliminate the foods that testing reveals you are allergic to. Or the doctor may cut from your diet the six foods most likely to cause allergies: nuts, fish and shellfish, eggs, wheat, soy, and milk. If your symptoms improve, the foods are reintroduced one at a time, one every two weeks, to see which foods cause symptoms to return. In one study, cutting the six foods for six weeks reduced symptoms in nearly everyone. As foods were reintroduced, wheat and milk were the most likely to trigger a return of symptoms. If these measures do not help, eosinophilic esophagitis often responds to a course of the steroid fluticasone (Flovent) taken orally.

Drug therapy

Nonstop advertising has acquainted most people with antacids, the least expensive treatment for heartburn. These work by reducing the acidity of refluxed material. But much more effective are the drugs known as proton-pump inhibitors (PPIs), such as omeprazole (Prilosec, Zegerid), and the H2 blockers, such as cimetidine (Tagamet) and ranitidine (Zantac). Some of these drugs are available over the counter. PPIs are more effective than either antacids or H2 blockers but tend to be more costly and may cause some unwanted side effects. In severe cases, physicians combine various antireflux drugs, such as over-the-counter antacids and H2 blockers, or PPIs and prokinetic drugs that increase gastric emptying. However, PPIs without additional medications are generally preferable to combinations.

Following are descriptions of the various reflux drugs in the order in which physicians typically recommend or prescribe their use. For more information on all these drugs, see the Appendix.

Heartburn or heart attack?

Don't ignore the possibility that chest pain may mean a heart attack instead of heartburn. Symptoms associated with GERD can mimic the pain of a myocardial infarction (heart attack) or angina (chest pain caused by diminished blood flow through the coronary arteries), especially when the sensation is constricting rather than burning in nature. It can be dangerous to assume that your chest pain is caused by reflux.

People with known reflux disease should always seek medical attention if they experience chest discomfort brought on by exercise, which may signal either angina or a heart attack. Paying attention to the nature, severity, frequency, and duration of your chest pain is key. If it's a severe, pressing, or squeezing discomfort, it may be a heart attack. And heart attack pain lasts awhile. If it goes away in five to 10 minutes, it's probably not a heart attack. It could be angina, however, which does require a visit to the doctor—and does require treatment. It's important not to dismiss chest tightness, especially if it follows physical exercise.

Proton-pump inhibitors

PPIs are more effective than H2 blockers for reducing gastric acid. PPIs work by inactivating a specific enzyme responsible for the final step of acid release in the stomach.

PPIs available over the counter include esomeprazole (Nexium), lansoprazole (Prevacid), pantoprazole (Protonix), and omeprazole (Prilosec, Zegerid). (Zegerid is an immediate-release medication, in contrast to other PPIs, which are delayed-release.) PPIs available only by prescription include rabeprazole (Aciphex) and dexlansoprazole (Dexilant). All these medications effectively heal esophagitis and alleviate heartburn.

In general, PPIs are considered safe medicines. But they may make the gastrointestinal tract more susceptible to bacterial infections—including a serious diarrheal disease called *Clostridium difficile*—and may increase the long-term risk of hip fractures. Also, you should avoid the PPIs omeprazole and esomeprazole if you are taking clopidogrel (Plavix), a drug that helps prevent blood clots. Those two PPIs reduce the effectiveness of clopidogrel, potentially placing you at a higher risk of heart attack or stroke.

Despite these concerns, PPIs are the preferred medication for treating esophagitis and severe cases of GERD. Doctors often recommend them first for frequent heartburn of all types. But once your symptoms recede, an H2 blocker also can be effective. If your symptoms respond to PPIs, the American Gastroenterological Association advises that you taper off the drugs to determine whether they can be stopped or, if not, to find the lowest effective dose, periodically re-evaluating the dose with your physician. The organization believes that some people, including those with Barrett's esophagus, need to stay on PPIs for the long term.

H2 blockers

For chronic reflux, histamine$_2$-receptor antagonists (H2 blockers) are now widely available either by prescription or, in smaller doses, over the counter. They are often effective for GERD symptoms that don't respond to antacids or changes in eating habits. They are also useful for long-term maintenance in some people who have responded initially to a PPI.

H2 blockers work by countering the effect of histamine (which stimulates gastric acid production), thereby decreasing the amount of acid that the stomach produces. They act directly on the stomach's acid-secreting cells to stop them from making hydrochloric acid, particularly at night when acid gathers in the stomach and can wash back into the esophagus. Cimetidine (Tagamet) was the first H2 blocker on the market. Others available in the United States include ranitidine

(Zantac), famotidine (Pepcid), and nizatidine (Axid).

Ranitidine has been reported to decrease the sensitivity of receptors in the esophagus to acid exposure, so H2 blockers may help for reflux hypersensitivity.

For people whose heartburn is troublesome only at night, a single dose of an H2 blocker taken at bedtime may suffice, but people whose symptoms occur during both day and night will need more frequent doses. All the H2 blockers are equally effective, so switching to another if one fails to work is likely to be fruitless. Increasing the dose, however, may be helpful.

H2 blockers are considered relatively safe, and side effects are infrequent.

Antacids

These inexpensive over-the-counter remedies neutralize digestive acids in the stomach and esophagus, at least in mild cases of heartburn. While many people find tablets more convenient, liquids provide faster relief. Tablets must be chewed thoroughly in order to be effective. The best time to take an antacid is after a meal or when symptoms occur. The usual recommended dosage is 1 to 2 tablespoons (or tablets) each time.

There are three basic salts used in antacids: magnesium, aluminum, and calcium. A major side effect of magnesium hydroxide is diarrhea, while the most common side effect of antacids containing aluminum hydroxide is constipation. Those high in calcium (Tums, Rolaids, Titralac, and Alka-2) are probably the strongest. Calcium carbonate products have been used for centuries in the form of chalk powder and ground oyster shell. However, they, too, can cause constipation if you use them often. Sodium bicarbonate, or baking soda, is less powerful than other antacids. It's the active ingredient in many seltzer antacids (Alka-Seltzer, Bromo-Seltzer) and is found in mineral water. You should avoid sodium if you have high blood pressure (hypertension) or heart failure.

Because no single agent is perfect, many antacids combine several ingredients that are designed to balance their respective side effects.

Prokinetic agents

Prokinetics—or gastrokinetics, as they're occasionally called—help empty the stomach of acids and fluids. They can also improve LES muscle tone. These medications are used only for occasional cases of GERD, either with or in place of H2 blockers, particularly when the stomach appears to empty slowly.

Antidepressants

As with many functional gastrointestinal disorders involving pain, various antidepressants are used to alter the activity of nerves involved in heartburn pain (see "Antidepressants to treat the body as well as the mind," page 34). Because the separation of heartburn types into the current categories is so recent, there are few studies to guide physicians on which type of antidepressant might work best for a particular pattern of symptoms and test results. In one study of people with reflux hypersensitivity, only 39% of participants reported continued heartburn symptoms after taking the SSRI antidepressant citalopram (Celexa) for six months, compared with 67% of people taking a placebo.

Herbal remedies

Some people find herbs and other natural remedies helpful in treating heartburn symptoms.

Chamomile. A cup of chamomile tea may have a soothing effect on the digestive tract. Avoid chamomile if you're allergic to ragweed.

Ginger. The root of the ginger plant is another well-known herbal digestive aid and has been a folk remedy for heartburn for centuries.

Licorice. This remedy has proved effective in several studies. Licorice is said to increase the mucous coating of the esophageal lining, helping it resist the irritating effects of stomach acid. Deglycyrrhizinated licorice, or DGL, is available in pill or liquid form. It is considered safe to take indefinitely.

Other natural remedies. A variety of other remedies have been used over the centuries, but not enough scientific studies have been done to confirm their effectiveness. Catnip, fennel, marshmallow root, and papaya tea have all been said to aid in digestion and act as a buffer to stop heartburn. Some people eat fresh papaya as a digestive aid. Others swear by raw potato juice, three times a day. However, these remedies have not been reviewed for safety or effectiveness by the FDA.

Surgical options for reflux

Medication and lifestyle changes can successfully control 95% of GERD cases, but for a few people, surgery is the best option. For example, surgery might be preferable for younger people who want to avoid taking PPIs over a period of many years. However, the relief provided by surgery might not be permanent, and medications might be necessary again at some point. Doctors might also suggest surgery for occasional cases of erosive esophagitis that do not improve with drug therapy, strictures that recur despite treatment, or uncommon instances of pneumonia or recurrent respiratory problems due to acid reflux that don't improve with drug therapy.

The goal of surgery is to tighten the LES. The operations are generally effective and can eliminate the need for all GERD medications for some time. However, surgical procedures are more likely to provide relief for people with erosive reflux disease than those with non-erosive disease.

Fundoplication

The most common antireflux operation is the Nissen (360-degree) fundoplication, also known as a stomach wrap. Nissen fundoplication involves grabbing a portion of the top of the stomach and looping it around the lower end of the esophagus and LES to create an artificial sphincter or pinch valve. This prevents stomach acid from surging upward into the esophagus (see Figure 6, below left). The wrap must be tight enough to prevent the acid from coming back up, but not so tight that food can't enter and a satisfying belch can't escape. Partial fundoplication, in which the stomach is wrapped only partway around the esophagus, is another option.

Figure 6: Surgery for GERD

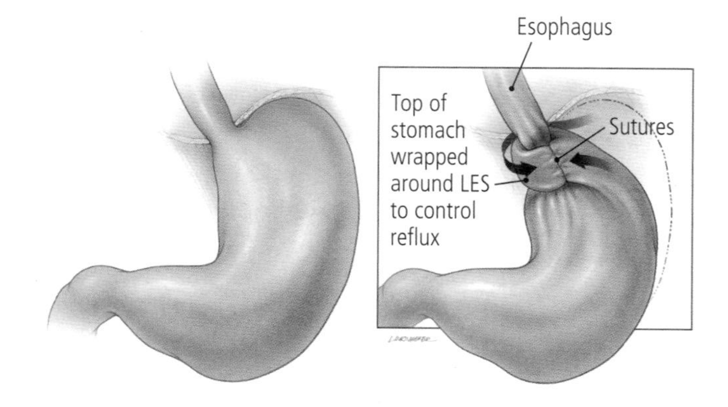

Most cases of GERD can be managed successfully with medications. But in a few cases, a surgical procedure called fundoplication is used to fold the top of the stomach around the lower end of the esophagus to create a high-pressure zone that functions as a lower esophageal sphincter.

Over time, however, the stomach wrap can loosen. When that happens, the person may need to resume medications and, in a small number of cases, undergo surgery to redo the procedure.

Today, most surgeons perform fundoplication as a laparoscopic procedure, in which miniature instruments and cameras are inserted into tiny incisions in the upper abdomen. This approach is associated with a shorter hospital stay and faster recovery.

Other procedures

A number of new procedures, known collectively as transoral incisionless fundoplication, rely on an endoscope (a tube that's placed down the throat) to reconstruct the LES and hold it tighter with tiny fasteners. The comparative risks, benefits, and long-term results of surgical and less-invasive endoscopic procedures to treat GERD are not clear, and your insurer may decline coverage for the endoscopic treatment. People with a large hiatal hernia that needs repair must have a surgical rather than endoscopic approach.

In 2012, the FDA approved use of a device for magnetic esophageal sphincter enhancement, called LINX, consisting of a ring of magnetic beads that is inserted laparoscopically and placed around the weak sphincter. The magnetic attraction keeps the ring tight enough to prevent reflux, but the sphincter can open as needed with the force of a swallow or belch. There are no long-term studies of this approach, and your insurer may consider the procedure investigational and decline coverage.

A different endoscopic approach, called Stretta, delivers radiofrequency energy to the sphincter muscle. As it heals, the muscle thickens and stiffens, reducing reflux. However, studies using the approach have had mixed results, and your insurer may consider the procedure investigational.

Dyspepsia

You're having trouble with your stomach. You feel uncomfortable. It's not heartburn, but it's related to eating. Sometimes the discomfort begins during a meal, sometimes about half an hour later. You feel bloated and full or have a burning pain. You're nauseated, and sometimes you even vomit. You might call it an "upset stomach" or "indigestion." Doctors call it dyspepsia—literally, "bad digestion." The word comes from the Greek *dys*, which means bad, and *peptein*, which means "to cook" or "to digest."

The problem can last for months, though it tends to come and go in spurts. Your first thought may be that you have developed an ulcer, or even cancer, but up to 60% of the time there is no identifiable cause for persistent upper abdominal pain or discomfort. The term for this is functional dyspepsia or non-ulcer dyspepsia.

Functional dyspepsia affects about a quarter of the population—twice as many as have ulcers—and it hits men and women equally. It's responsible for a significant proportion of visits to primary care doctors. Not only is the cause of functional dyspepsia unknown, but even more frustrating, there's no surefire cure.

Figure 7: How an ulcer starts

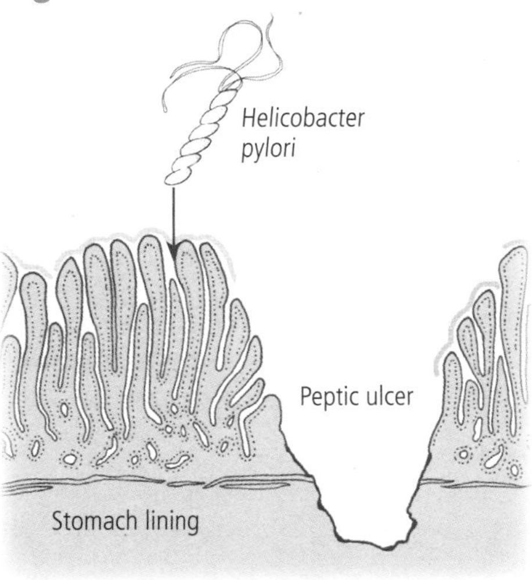

In the early 1980s, researchers identified a major culprit in ulcers—the corkscrew-shaped bacterium *Helicobacter pylori*. It attaches to the surface of the stomach by twisting through the mucus that protects the stomach lining from corrosive gastric juices. Up to 90% of people with duodenal ulcers and 75% to 85% of those with gastric (stomach) ulcers are infected with *H. pylori*.

The other major cause of ulcers is the use of NSAIDs, such as aspirin and ibuprofen.

Causes of dyspepsia

Peptic ulcers—that is, ulcers in either the stomach or the duodenum (the upper small intestine)—are one common cause of dyspepsia. About 10% of Americans develop a peptic ulcer at some point.

Peptic ulcers are raw, crater-like breaks in the mucosal lining of the digestive tract (see Figure 7, at left). They are generally circular and rarely more than an inch in diameter. They are linked to the erosive action of gastric acid and sometimes to a reduction in protective mucus. In essence, the stomach, which is designed to digest foods, is digesting a part of its own lining.

The most common cause of peptic ulcers is infection with the bacterium *Helicobacter pylori*. Other causes include irritating substances such as aspirin, ibuprofen, and other nonsteroidal anti-inflammatory drugs (NSAIDs). Cigarette smoking impairs the healing of ulcers, and stress appears to aggravate ulcer symptoms. Studies show there's also a genetic component, as ulcers sometimes run in families. They occur more often in people with type O blood than in those with other blood types. Sometimes there is no known cause (a condition called idiopathic ulcer).

Besides ulcers, other identifiable causes of dyspepsia include gastroesophageal reflux disease and certain types of gastritis (inflammation of the stomach). Less commonly, gallstones and even some serious conditions such as stomach cancer or angina may cause dyspepsia (see "What else could it be?" on page 16).

Functional dyspepsia

When common tests can't identify a cause, the problem is said to be functional dyspepsia. Many experts doubt that excess gastric acid is to blame for this perplexing

What else could it be?

At least some of the distress associated with functional dyspepsia reflects the fear that a more serious condition may be going undetected. This is rarely the case, especially when symptoms persist for months or years without worsening. Fortunately, more serious ailments have characteristics that set them apart from functional dyspepsia.

Gallstones. Stones can dwell silently in the gallbladder or can produce painful attacks—typically after a large, high-fat meal—if the gallbladder contracts and a stone lodges in its neck. The pain is usually located just under the right rib cage or in the upper middle abdomen and may radiate to the right shoulder or back. Attacks of pain due to gallstones are generally infrequent—often only several times a year and frequently less than that.

Stomach cancer. Malignancies of the stomach generally occur later in life, after age 50. Tumors that burrow into the stomach wall often produce symptoms that resemble those associated with ulcers. The pain is often brought on by eating. Consuming a full meal can become impossible if growths protrude into the hollow of the organ or spread through the stomach wall, making it too stiff to expand. Warning signs include bleeding, persistent vomiting, a constant sense of nausea or fullness that interferes with normal eating, and weight loss. Treatment of stomach cancer usually requires the surgical removal of all or part of the stomach.

Angina. This pain and tightness, which occurs when not enough blood is getting to your heart muscle, may feel like heartburn or dyspepsia (see "Heartburn or heart attack?" on page 12). It is felt in the mid-chest and typically occurs with exertion. If angina is a possibility, cardiac tests such as an electrocardiogram, stress test, echocardiogram, or imaging of the coronary arteries may be required.

Figure 8: Other causes of pain

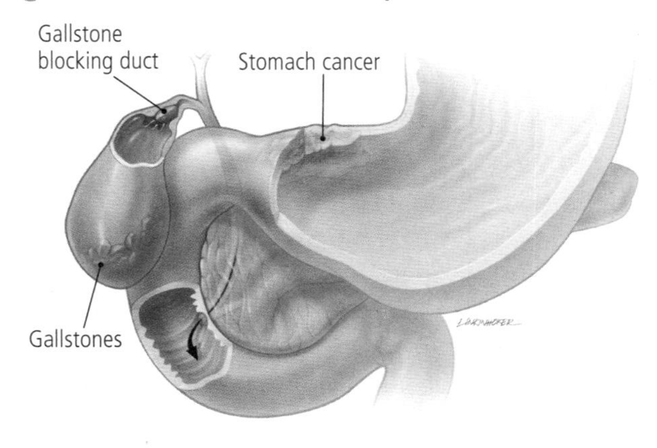

Gallstones can cause pain and inflammation if they block the neck of the gallbladder or the bile duct (rather than passing into the small intestine, as shown by the arrow). Cancer of the stomach lining can create a sensation of painful bloating. Angina (not shown) is the result of inadequate blood supply to the heart.

problem. Studies have found no irregularities in acid secretion in people with dyspepsia and no correlation between symptoms and increased acid production. But the theory remains under consideration, as does the possibility that the abdominal pain associated with functional dyspepsia results from some alteration that increases the sensitivity of the gastric or duodenal mucosa to acid. Following are some other ideas:

Pain hypersensitivity. Many experts believe that people with functional dyspepsia are more sensitive to pain than other people are, and that they may have a lower threshold for pain than their healthy counterparts. Symptoms may result from excessive sensitivity of the stomach to distension or other stimuli.

Motility problems. The symptoms of functional dyspepsia may reflect abnormal motility—that is, a problem with the movement of the digestive tract, which might slow the emptying of the stomach, triggering symptoms.

Stress, anxiety, or other psychological factors. Anxiety and emotional stress or depression are common in people with functional dyspepsia. Treating the underlying discomfort improves the psychological distress for some people, while in other cases, removing stressful feelings may improve the stomach discomfort.

***H. pylori* infection.** While the role of *H. pylori* in ulcers and gastritis is well established, its involvement in functional dyspepsia is less clear. *H. pylori* infection is only slightly more common in people with functional dyspepsia than in others. In most cases, eradicating *H. pylori* with antibiotics doesn't significantly improve functional dyspepsia symptoms.

Evaluating dyspepsia

During a medical exam, your doctor will ask for details about your symptoms, including how long and how often they have been occurring, exactly where you feel the discomfort, how severe the pain is, and how the timing and content of your meals and snacks seems to alter your symptoms. One immediate suspect will likely be ulcers. Aside from dyspepsia, "alarm" symptoms that may point to an ulcer include

- evidence of bleeding, such as passing black stools or vomiting blood or material that resembles coffee grounds
- repeatedly vomiting large amounts of sour juice and food, which can signal an obstructing ulcer
- sudden, overwhelming pain—a rare but frightening signal that the ulcer has perforated the stomach or duodenal wall.

Discomfort that feels worse on an empty stomach and is relieved by eating suggests a duodenal ulcer, although the diagnosis isn't definitive without further testing. Ulcer pain may wake you during the night. If this pain is relieved by antacids, H2 blockers, or proton-pump inhibitors (PPIs) taken at bedtime, it might indicate an ulcer. Your physician will also address other health habits, such as whether you smoke or drink alcoholic beverages, and will want to know if other family members have ever been diagnosed with an ulcer.

As a first step toward both diagnosis and treatment, your doctor will inquire about your use of NSAIDs and probably order a fecal, blood, or breath test to detect *H. pylori* bacteria, which can cause stomach inflammation in addition to ulcers. If the test is positive, the doctor will prescribe antibiotics to eradicate the bacteria. If the test is negative, or if your symptoms don't improve after antibiotic treatment, your doctor will likely prescribe one or more drugs that curtail acid secretion to see if the dyspepsia clears. If symptoms have not improved after a few weeks, the next step will likely be an endoscopy to check for an ulcer (see Figure 9, above right).

Do you have functional dyspepsia?

The Rome IV criteria specify functional dyspepsia must include one or more of the following for the past three months, with symptoms beginning at least six months before diagnosis:

- ✔ bothersome feeling of fullness after eating
- ✔ early feeling of fullness
- ✔ pain in the upper abdomen
- ✔ burning in the upper abdomen.

There must also be no evidence of structural disease (including any seen with upper GI endoscopy; see Figure 9, above right) that is likely to explain the symptoms.

Figure 9: Upper GI endoscopy

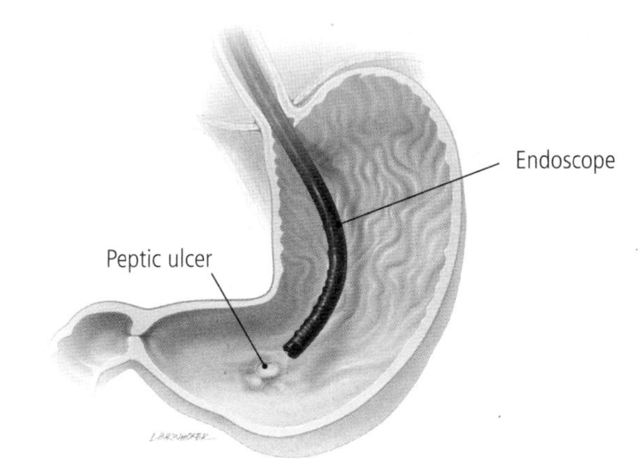

An endoscope is a flexible tube with a light and camera at the end that a doctor uses to view the interior of a person's esophagus and stomach. During this procedure, the person lies on his or her side as the doctor gently slides the scope through the mouth and down the esophagus into the stomach, while watching for lesions on a video monitor.

Endoscopy is an outpatient test that is highly accurate for finding ulcers. It should not be ordered, however, if a perforation is suspected; in that case a CT scan is usually the test of choice, and emergency surgery may be necessary.

Occasionally, there is a serious underlying cause for dyspepsia, such as stomach cancer (see "What else could it be?" on page 16). People ages 60 and over (some experts say 50 or 55 and over) with new dyspepsia and those with a family history of gastrointestinal cancers should have an endoscopy right away to look for cancer. Additional worrisome symptoms, such as weight loss, dysphagia (difficulty swallowing), gastrointestinal bleeding, or anemia (low red blood cell count), may also warrant immediate attention.

Diagnosing functional dyspepsia

If no cause of the abdominal discomfort is identified, the doctor may conclude that the symptoms are due to functional dyspepsia, since functional dyspepsia and ulcers share many of the same features. Both conditions seem to be stress-related and affect people of all ages. In many cases, the symptoms of both respond to treatment with a placebo. In both conditions, pressing on the person's abdomen can produce tenderness.

Although the cause of functional dyspepsia is not known, various factors may contribute:

Duodenitis. Long-term inflammation of the lining of the duodenum—called duodenitis—may produce symptoms of functional dyspepsia. However, less than 20% of people with functional dyspepsia have this condition.

Diet. Up to 80% of people with functional dyspepsia report that eating fatty foods brings on their symptoms. This connection makes sense because fat ingestion not only delays gastric emptying but also increases distension of the stomach. Substances like alcohol and coffee may also aggravate symptoms.

Drugs. NSAIDs, especially aspirin, can cause dyspepsia, ulcers, and gastritis. Other drugs such as opioids, iron preparations, and digitalis may also cause dyspepsia.

Treating dyspepsia

Ulcers are generally treated with PPIs to reduce stomach acid and with combinations of antibiotics to eliminate *H. pylori* infection, if it is present. Because NSAIDs often cause gastric irritation, you should stop taking them, if possible. Although PPIs are generally given for only eight to 12 weeks, you might take them for longer if you need to keep using an NSAID. You will probably have another endoscopy after eight to 12 weeks on a PPI to confirm that the ulcer has healed and is not a cancer.

For functional dyspepsia, there is no truly effective drug. However, doctors often recommend over-the-counter antacids, H2 blockers, and omeprazole (Prilosec OTC). In one study, people with functional dyspepsia and without depression were more likely to improve when treated with the tricyclic antidepressant amitriptyline (Elavil, Endep)—but with doses much smaller than those used for depression—than when given an SSRI antidepressant or a placebo. Tricyclic antidepressants are thought to reduce the sensitivity of the stomach to painful stimuli, such as distension. Medications that improve gastric emptying, such as metoclopramide (Reglan), have been used for a few weeks, with cautions about serious neurological side effects that can occur, but these drugs are not generally effective for functional dyspepsia.

Anticholinergic medications that relax muscles in the digestive tract, such as hyoscyamine (Levsin), may be used for up to four to six weeks. Simethicone, which rids the gut of gas bubbles, is safe and may help if you have both functional dyspepsia and flatulence.

Herbal remedies may also be worth a try. In several clinical trials, a combination of enteric-coated capsules of peppermint oil and caraway oil successfully reduced fullness, bloating, and gastrointestinal spasms in people with functional dyspepsia. (Enteric-coated means that the preparation is able to pass through the stomach and won't dissolve until it reaches the small intestine.) Be aware, however, that peppermint oil may trigger reflux in people who are predisposed to it.

Finally, there are many lifestyle changes that can help (see "Lifestyle modifications for functional dyspepsia," at left). In fact, many people prefer lifestyle changes over long-term medication use because of the overall improvement in well-being they experience.

Lifestyle modifications for functional dyspepsia

Body position, diet, exercise habits, and adequate sleep can help.

Make good eating choices

- Avoid foods that trigger symptoms. Common triggers are caffeine, chocolate, alcohol, and spicy, acidic, or fatty foods.
- Eat smaller, more frequent meals so your stomach does not become distended and empties more quickly.
- Chew your food slowly and completely.
- Avoid activities that result in swallowing excess air, such as smoking, eating quickly, chewing gum, and drinking carbonated beverages.
- Don't lie down within two hours of eating.
- Keep your weight under control.

Reduce stress

- Use stress reduction techniques, including relaxation therapies.
- Exercise. (In addition to being good for your overall health, it's a proven stress reducer.)
- Try cognitive behavioral therapy.

Reduce fatigue

- Get enough rest.
- Go to bed and get up at the same times each day.
- Avoid caffeine after noon.

Exercise

- Perform aerobic exercise three to five times a week for 20 to 40 minutes per session.
- Don't exercise immediately after eating.

Irritable bowel syndrome

Another common intestinal disorder with a myriad of unpleasant symptoms is irritable bowel syndrome (IBS). IBS affects millions of people, but its cause is unclear—meaning that by definition it is a functional ailment. Equally frustrating, treatment is often a trial-and-error process that may or may not be successful. It is the most common diagnosis made by gastroenterologists and accounts for as many as 3.5 million physician visits and 2.2 million prescriptions per year. Yet IBS may well be the most challenging functional gastrointestinal disorder, for doctors and their patients alike. Several studies have found that people with IBS have a significantly lower quality of life than people without the syndrome and that IBS generally underdiagnosed.

Through the years, IBS has been called by many names—spastic colon, spastic bowel, colitis, mucous colitis, and functional bowel disease. None of these names is quite accurate.

Do you have IBS?

According to the Rome IV criteria, you have IBS if you have had recurrent abdominal pain at least one day per week in the past three months, beginning at least six months ago, and two or more of the following statements apply:

- ✔ The pain is related to defecation (may improve or worsen after a bowel movement).
- ✔ The pain is associated with a change in the frequency of bowel movements.
- ✔ The stool itself looks different (harder or looser than usual).

Tracking and reporting the following symptoms will help your physician make the diagnosis and identify what type of IBS you have:

- ✔ abnormal stool frequency (more than three bowel movements per day or less than three per week)
- ✔ abnormal stool form (hard or loose stool) more than one in every four times
- ✔ abnormal stool passage (straining, urgency, or the feeling of incomplete evacuation) more than one in four times
- ✔ passage of mucus in more than one in every four bowel movements
- ✔ bloating or the sensation of having a distended abdomen on more than one out of every four days.

What is IBS?

IBS usually begins in the late teens, 20s, or 30s. You're a relatively healthy person; then one day you begin to suffer intermittent cramps in the lower abdomen. You have to move your bowels more often than usual, and when you have to go, you have to get to a toilet right away. Your stools are loose and watery, possibly containing mucus. Sometimes, you feel bloated and full of gas.

After a while, the cramps return, but this time when you try to go to the bathroom, nothing happens. You're constipated. And back and forth it goes—diarrhea, then constipation, and pain and bloating in between. Or instead of alternating between constipation and diarrhea, you always have one without the other (but always with at least some abdominal pain). Irritable bowel syndrome is the catchall term for this mixed bag of symptoms.

It's a common disorder, with no known cause. The most frequently reported symptom is pain or discomfort in the abdomen. People with IBS may feel the pain subside after a bowel movement or passing gas. But they also may feel that they haven't fully emptied their rectum after a movement.

A survey of 3,254 adults who met the criteria for IBS summarized some of the reasons why this condition can be so aggravating. Among other things, the survey found that

- the diagnosis was typically made four years after the start of IBS symptoms
- 77% of respondents had tried over-the-counter remedies (three to four different products, on average) before discussing their symptoms with a doctor

Continued on page 21

What else could it be, if it isn't IBS?

A number of gastrointestinal diseases can cause symptoms similar to those of IBS.

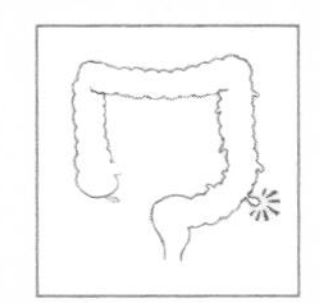

Diverticular disease. Small sacs or pouches—known as diverticula—may bulge through the colon's inner lining, where the blood vessels enter the colon, piercing its walls and causing areas of weakness. Although this is most common after age 50, younger people occasionally develop diverticula. The existence of such pouches is a condition known as diverticulosis. However, when a diverticulum becomes inflamed or infected, the condition is called diverticulitis. The symptoms of diverticulitis are generally much more intense than those of IBS and may include severe pain in the lower left part of the abdomen, chills, fever, and an elevated white blood cell count.

Treatment of diverticulitis involves a liquid diet to let the bowel rest and antibiotic therapy to clear the infection (although in the mildest cases, antibiotics might not be necessary). After the immediate inflammation has stabilized, people switch to a steady high-fiber diet to help prevent flare-ups. Although people with diverticulosis are often advised to avoid nuts and seeds, there is no scientific support for this recommendation. Surgery may be required when diverticulitis is complicated (for example, by an abscess, a collection of pus) or recurrent.

Inflammatory bowel disease (IBD). This condition is characterized by chronic inflammation of a segment or segments of the gastrointestinal tract. The precise cause is not known. The two main types of IBD are Crohn's disease and ulcerative colitis. The two often have similar symptoms and are treated in similar ways, yet physicians regard them as distinct. IBD has a wide variety of symptoms, including persistent abdominal pain, diarrhea, rectal bleeding, fever, and weight loss.

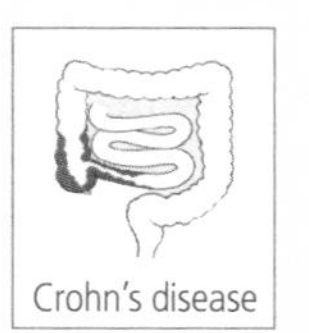
Crohn's disease

- **Crohn's disease,** a type of IBD, can occur anywhere in the digestive tract, from the mouth to the anus, but it's usually found at the end of the small intestine (ileum), in the colon, or both. The bowel wall becomes thickened as well as constantly inflamed, and leakage of intestinal contents from the bowel can cause internal abscesses. Another complication is a fistula (an abnormal passage) that allows intestinal material to pass through the wall of the intestine into another segment of the intestine or another organ and that may require surgery. Severe bleeding is not likely with Crohn's disease.

  Crohn's disease usually appears in young people, who develop pain in the right side of the abdomen, a low-grade fever, and perhaps changes in bowel movements. Some people develop a fistula or abscess around the anus.

  In some cases, surgery is needed to treat a complication of the disease, such as bowel obstruction. About 40% to 60% of those with Crohn's eventually need surgery to remove damaged areas of their small intestine or colon.

- **Ulcerative colitis,** the other principal type of IBD, is characterized by inflammation limited to the lining, or mucosa, of the colon. Like IBS, it can cause lower abdominal pain and diarrhea. Unlike IBS, the stool generally contains blood, and bowel symptoms may be accompanied by fever, weight loss, an elevated white blood cell count, and a variety of skin lesions and arthritis. Ulcerative colitis is easier to diagnose than Crohn's disease and is treated with many of the same medications.

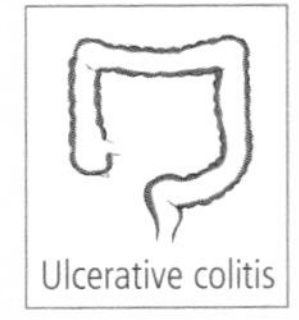
Ulcerative colitis

Medications that control inflammation can help relieve IBD symptoms. The drugs used most commonly are aminosalicylates (cousins of aspirin); corticosteroids (potent anti-inflammatory agents), such as prednisone and budesonide; and immunosuppressants and antibiotics. For those who don't respond to standard treatments, biologic agents block the action of inflammatory proteins. These include adalimumab (Humira), infliximab (Remicade), and vedolizumab (Entyvio), approved for both types of IBD, and certolizumab pegol (Cimzia), natalizumab (Tysabri), and ustekinumab (Stelara), which are approved only for certain patients with Crohn's disease. More of these agents are likely to be approved through an FDA program that fast-tracks products that are biologically similar to, or interchangeable with, approved biologics.

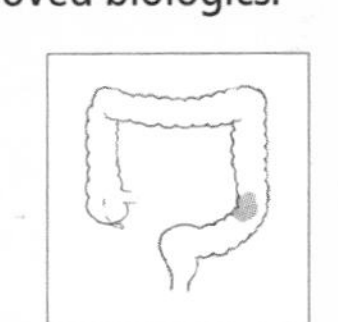

Colorectal cancer. Colorectal cancer is the third most common form of cancer in both men and women, with an estimated 154,000 new cases diagnosed in the United States each year. Early on, colon cancer causes no symptoms. Later, its symptoms can be similar to those of IBS—abdominal pain, cramping, bloating, gas pains, and a change in bowel patterns. In addition, blood in the stool or rectal bleeding is often present. Advanced cancer is likely to cause bloody bowel movements, severe constipation if the intestine is obstructed, and weight loss. Thus, it's vital to get checked without delay should these symptoms occur.

The good news is that most cases of colon cancer can be prevented through screening (see Table 2, page 21). Almost all precancerous growths (polyps) can be spotted and removed during a colonoscopy. Early-stage, localized colon cancers are curable by surgery in 90% of cases.

Celiac disease. Also known as celiac sprue, celiac disease is a genetically based disorder that damages the small intestine and may result in mild to severe symptoms. As many as one million Americans have the disease, which clusters in families, primarily occurring in whites of European ancestry.

When people with celiac disease eat foods containing gluten—a protein found in wheat, rye, and barley—their immune systems attack the gluten, and in the process, they also flatten the villi, tiny finger-like projections lining the small intestine that help the body absorb nutrients. A simple blood test for higher-than-normal levels of antibodies is the first step in diagnosing the disease. If the test is positive, a biopsy of the small intestine, performed through a standard endoscope, can confirm the diagnosis. Treatment is straightforward: a gluten-free diet. Symptoms often improve within days, and the small intestine gradually returns to normal function.

Continued from page 19

- on average, they missed school or work two days per month and worked with diminished productivity another nine days per month because of IBS symptoms
- only 26% of participants were very satisfied with the FDA-approved prescription medications for the conditions.

All in all, too many people are suffering from this perplexing condition. If you have some of the symptoms of IBS, you may want to try some of the lifestyle changes in this report to see if they help you feel better. However, if you are truly miserable or have symptoms (such as unexplained weight loss, rectal bleeding, or abdominal pain during the night) that make you worry about the possibility of more serious illness, don't wait to seek medical attention (see "What else could it be, if it isn't IBS?" on page 20).

While some people with IBS have daily episodes or continuous symptoms, others experience long symptom-free periods. These patterns make it hard to know whether someone has IBS or an occasional difficulty that's part of the bowel's normal response to stress or diet. Whether to label the symptoms as IBS usually depends on their frequency and duration: current criteria for this diagnosis are abdominal pain and changed bowel habits at least one day per week for at least three months.

IBS has no clearly identified organic basis—that is, there's no physical abnormality or disease at the root of the problem. And doctors don't regard IBS as a forerunner of more serious diseases, such as ulcerative colitis, Crohn's disease, colon cancer, or stomach cancer.

Possible causes of IBS

IBS is probably not a single disease, but rather a set of symptoms that stem from a variety of causes. It may be generally described as a disorder in the functioning of the gastrointestinal tract. Some experts suspect that IBS involves disturbances in the nerves or muscles in the gut. Others believe that abnormal processing of gut sensations in the brain may hold the key, at least in some cases. The following are widely believed to be contributing causes.

Genetics

Nationwide studies in Sweden have shown that relatives of patients with IBS have a higher risk of the disorder, with the closest relatives having the highest risk. In addition, some studies have identified specific genetic changes that may underlie IBS in some people.

Table 2: Guidelines for colorectal cancer screening

Symptoms of IBS can be similar to those of colorectal cancer. Follow these guidelines for screening. Note that these screening recommendations are for people who have no symptoms of colorectal cancer. If you have symptoms that suggest colorectal cancer, such as blood in the stool, you should undergo diagnostic testing. Some guidelines recommend that people older than 75 or who are likely to die within 10 years from another health problem and have never had colon cancer or polyps in prior screenings should not undergo further screening for colon cancer.

YOUR RISK CATEGORY	SCREENING RECOMMENDATION
Average risk: Age 50 or older without any of the risk factors noted below. In 2018, the American Cancer Society lowered its recommended starting age to 45.	One of the following is recommended: • colonoscopy every 10 years • flexible sigmoidoscopy every five years • fecal occult blood test with three samples from separate stools every year • computed tomography (CT) colonography (virtual colonoscopy) every five years • fecal DNA test every three years.
Moderate risk: Family history of colorectal cancer in a first-degree relative (parent, sibling, or child)	Colonoscopy every five years beginning at age 40, or starting 10 years younger than the age at diagnosis of the person's youngest affected relative (whichever is younger).
Moderate risk: Personal history of colorectal cancer	Colonoscopy: Consult your doctor for frequency guidelines based on your personal health risks.
High risk: Certain genetic and disease characteristics; consult your doctor about your specific risk factors	Colonoscopy (or flexible sigmoidoscopy in some cases) beginning in adolescence or early adulthood, depending on your personal and family health history.

Source: Screening for Colorectal Cancer: A Guidance Statement from the American College of Physicians, 2012.

Infection

Several studies have demonstrated that a bout of infectious gastroenteritis (stomach or bowel inflammation, often resulting from a foodborne infection) may be a major factor in causing IBS. In a 2017 analysis of studies involving 21,421 people with infectious gastroenteritis (caused by viruses, bacteria, or other microorganisms), the risk of developing IBS in the next 12 months was about 10%—more than four times higher than in people who had not had food poisoning or other infectious gastroenteritis. Gastroenteritis caused by protozoa or parasites was the most likely to be followed by IBS, with 41.9% of people affected. Those at highest risk of developing IBS after an infection were women, people with the most severe infections, those who received antibiotic therapy, and those who experienced psychological distress at the time of the infection.

Overgrowth of intestinal bacteria

Another possible explanation for IBS is the overgrowth of bacteria in the small intestine. A certain amount of bacteria normally live there, but in this case the numbers are greater and the species are similar to those that usually reside in the colon. This overgrowth may cause the feeling of bloating and the passing of excess gas that are common symptoms of IBS. Researchers have found some evidence of bacterial overgrowth in the small intestines of people with IBS, and it appears that bacterial overgrowth may contribute to many common symptoms of IBS, including bloating and distension, diarrhea, constipation, and heightened sensitivity to pain. Treatment with antibiotics may improve some of these symptoms (see "Medications for IBS," page 26). Treatment with probiotics, live microbes intended to confer health benefits (see "Probiotics and prebiotics," page 28), provides relief for some people with IBS, but there is currently no way to identify who is most likely to benefit.

Colon activity

Because the cramping pain associated with IBS is perceived by patients as coming from the colon, researchers have concentrated on this part of the gastrointestinal tract, searching for any irregularities. So far, the findings have been inconsistent.

Some researchers have found that the colon muscle of a person with IBS begins to spasm after only mild stimulation (such as distension due to stool or gas). The colon seems to be more sensitive than usual, so it responds strongly to stimuli that wouldn't affect other people. Sometimes, the spasms lead to diarrhea; other times, to constipation. But some studies show that most of the time, colonic motor activity is no different for people with IBS than for anyone else.

Heightened sensitivity

Another possible explanation for these bothersome symptoms is that people with IBS have a heightened awareness of the inner workings of their gut. In several well-known experiments, balloons were inflated in the sigmoid colon, rectum, and small intestine of subjects. Those with IBS generally had a much lower threshold for experiencing pain than the healthy volunteers. Scientists believe that this lower pain threshold may be related to the dispatch of nerve signals from gut to brain.

Hormonal factors

Hormones produced in the gastrointestinal tract, such as cholecystokinin and motilin, have also been suspected of triggering IBS symptoms through their effects on bowel motility, but studies have not been definitive. Women with IBS often have more symptoms during their menstrual periods, suggesting that changes in the levels of reproductive hormones can increase IBS symptoms.

Dietary factors

In recent years, the understanding of foods that can trigger IBS symptoms has expanded greatly. For some people, certain sugar-like molecules found in many foods—including milk, some fruits and vegetables, wheat, rye, high-fructose corn syrup, and artificial sweeteners—can be difficult to digest. Gut bacteria feed on these sugars, creating the gas and bloating that's a hallmark of IBS. The problematic substances are known collectively as FODMAPs—short for fermentable oligosaccharides, disaccharides, monosaccharides, and polyols. A diet that avoids these troublesome sugars has garnered attention in recent years for use in IBS treatment (see

"Should you stop eating FODMAPs?" on page 25).

Other food triggers work in different ways to cause IBS symptoms. Caffeine causes loose stools in many people, but is more likely to affect those with IBS. Chocolate, dairy products, or large amounts of alcohol trigger spasms in some people. Sometimes the spasm delays the passage of stool, leading to constipation.

Some people simply can't tolerate certain dietary substances—for example, lactose (a sugar found in milk), fructose (a sugar found in fruit and used as a sweetener), or sorbitol (an artificial sweetener)—and develop bloating and diarrhea as a result. They may lack the ability to absorb one or more of these nutrients. Lactose intolerance is distinct from IBS, but the symptoms can overlap (see "Understanding food intolerance and food allergies," page 27), and the condition is common enough that your doctor may recommend that you eliminate lactose temporarily to see if your symptoms improve.

Bran and wheat flour may increase IBS symptoms (although sourdough bread might not). Gas-promoting vegetables such as beans and broccoli may contribute to bloating, as can excess fiber. On the other hand, some believe that a lack of dietary fiber may contribute to IBS. Fat in any form (animal or vegetable) is a strong stimulus of colon contractions, which can lead to pain, diarrhea, or constipation after a meal and can also contribute to IBS symptoms.

It's often a matter of trial and error to determine which foods trigger your symptoms. Try eliminating one food at a time to see which ones give you trouble. Keeping a food diary in which you record the foods that you eat as well as any IBS symptoms can also help.

Medications

Sorbitol, often found in cough medicine, can worsen diarrhea. SSRI antidepressants may worsen diarrhea, while tricyclic antidepressants may worsen constipation.

Stress and emotion

Stress is known to stimulate colon spasms in people with IBS. The process is not completely understood, but scientists point out that the intestines are controlled partly by the nervous system (see "The stress connection," page 30). Some studies have shown significantly higher stress levels among people with IBS compared with healthy individuals. And stress reduction, relaxation training, and counseling have each helped relieve IBS symptoms in some people.

Other emotional factors may also play a role. Studies have found considerably higher rates of psychiatric problems among people with IBS who see a specialist than among healthy people or those with structural bowel diseases.

One possible link between emotional disturbances and IBS relates to the neurotransmitter serotonin. Neurotransmitters are chemicals that convey messages between nerve cells. Like the brain, the gut produces serotonin, which in turn acts on nerves in the digestive tract. Some research suggests that people with IBS who suffer mainly from diarrhea may have higher levels of serotonin in the gut, while those with constipation-predominant IBS have lower levels.

Diagnosing IBS

Because there are no specific tests for IBS, the condition must be diagnosed based on symptoms and by process of elimination, sometimes with the use of tests to rule out other conditions. Fortunately, a diagnosis usually can be made with a single visit to a doctor.

The doctor takes a complete medical history, including a careful description of your symptoms. A physical exam and some routine laboratory tests are likely to be part of the evaluation, and a stool sample is useful to check for bleeding. Because diagnostic tests cannot confirm IBS but are used only to exclude other

Foods that may trigger IBS symptoms

- Caffeine
- Chewing gum, beverages, or foods sweetened with sorbitol or xylitol
- Chocolate
- Dairy products
- Fatty foods
- Gas-producing foods, such as broccoli, cabbage, beans, and onions
- Margarine
- Nuts
- Orange and grapefruit juices
- Other foods that are high in FODMAPs (see "Should you stop eating FODMAPs?" on page 25).

possible causes of symptoms, the goal is to use as few costly, invasive tests as possible. To accomplish this, experts in the treatment of gastrointestinal illnesses have developed a set of criteria to help identify people with IBS (see "Do you have IBS?" on page 19).

The doctor will also ask whether your symptoms started after an episode of gastroenteritis, or if they seem to be triggered by specific foods or medications, particularly milk products (which would suggest lactose intolerance) or foods and beverages that contain fructose or sorbitol. You may need to keep a food diary for a few weeks to help identify foods that provoke symptoms (see "Dietary factors," page 22).

It's especially important to consider emotional and psychological triggers. The doctor will want to know what prompted the visit and will ask about your lifestyle and stress level. It's not unusual for a traumatic life event such as divorce or the loss of a job to wreak havoc on the bowels and the psyche.

Other symptoms that accompany the pain may offer clues. If you have pain in your lower abdomen and a change in bowel movements, there may be an abnormality in the large intestine. A combination of abdominal pain and fever can signal inflammation (for example, diverticulitis), which requires immediate medical attention.

Another major diagnostic clue is bleeding from the digestive tract. People with IBS can have rectal bleeding, but IBS does not cause this bleeding. Instead, it reflects another cause, such as hemorrhoids. In general, bright red blood comes from the lower digestive tract, while black, tarry blood comes from the upper gastrointestinal tract. If you have bleeding, more tests must be performed to determine the cause.

During the physical exam, the physician will look for tenderness in your abdomen. If the tenderness is located in the lower right part, it may signal ileitis or appendicitis. Tenderness in the upper right part might come from gallstones and inflammation of the gallbladder. The doctor will also check for a mass, which might be a tumor, a large cyst, or impacted stool. If you have IBS, the physical exam will usually not reveal anything other than perhaps a mildly tender abdomen. A digital rectal exam is also usually part of the evaluation to check for masses in the rectum and, in men, the prostate. If your doctor suspects that you might have a serious disorder, he or she will order more tests.

Diagnostic tests

An experienced gastroenterologist will probably be able to make a preliminary determination as to whether IBS is the problem after hearing your initial story, even before ordering any tests. If tests are necessary to rule out other causes of symptoms, they may include a complete blood count, thyroid tests, and a measurement of erythrocyte sedimentation rate (ESR). The ESR, which gauges the speed at which mature red blood cells settle in a test tube, can be used to screen for inflammatory disease. You probably won't need further tests if your blood tests and your temperature are normal, there's no evidence of bleeding from the gastrointestinal tract, you're under age 50, and your symptoms are typical of IBS.

If you have persistent diarrhea, your doctor will have your stool samples examined for infectious agents, including intestinal parasites. Occasionally, the doctor may arrange for a stool collection to check for excess fecal fat content or weight, which would suggest that IBS is not the diagnosis.

A hydrogen breath test can help show whether your IBS symptoms are caused by an inability to properly absorb certain carbohydrates (see "Should you stop eating FODMAPs?" on page 25) or an overgrowth of bacteria in the small intestine. For this test, you blow up a balloon to provide a breath sample before you drink a solution containing a specific carbohydrate. After drinking the solution, you blow up the balloon again to provide another breath sample. The lab measures the hydrogen levels (which are usually minimal) in the two samples. The results can suggest whether antibiotics or specific food restrictions may ease the symptoms. If there's a chance that an inflammatory disease is causing your symptoms, your doctor may order a noninvasive stool test to detect calprotectin, a protein that is elevated in inflammatory disorders such as Crohn's disease and ulcerative colitis.

A person's age or atypical symptoms may persuade the doctor to conduct additional—and sometimes more invasive and expensive—diagnostic procedures.

Should you stop eating FODMAPs?

In 2001, an Australian dietitian named Sue Shepherd developed a diet that restricts foods high in FODMAPs. Today, growing evidence suggests that this low-FODMAP diet may tame IBS symptoms better than standard dietary advice for IBS. A 2017 study in *Clinical Gastroenterology and Hepatology* compared symptoms and quality of life in 45 people with IBS and diarrhea who followed a low-FODMAP diet and 39 others who were given common dietary advice for IBS but not specific FODMAP exclusions. After four weeks, both groups improved, but those on the low-FODMAP diet had greater improvement in IBS symptoms, such as pain and bloating. They also became less anxious, and IBS symptoms interfered less with their activities and quality of life.

Foods to avoid on the diet include

- high-FODMAP fruits, such as apples, stone fruits, and blackberries
- high-FODMAP vegetables, such as garlic, asparagus, and artichokes
- high-FODMAP legumes, such as red kidney beans and lima beans
- high-FODMAP bread and cereal products, such as those containing wheat, rye, or barley
- high-FODMAP dairy products, such as milk and yogurt
- high-FODMAP sweeteners such as high-fructose corn syrup and honey.

Does this mean that people with IBS and diarrhea should give up FODMAPs forever? No. The low-FODMAP diet is not meant to be permanent; nor is it an absolute restriction on FODMAPs. Rather, it is a three-step program to determine which, if any, of these carbohydrates are causing your symptoms, and to use that information to create the least restrictive diet possible. First, FODMAPs are eliminated for two to four weeks to see if symptoms improve. Next, if symptoms do show improvement, individual FODMAPs are reintroduced to see which ones you react to. After that is determined, the dietician can help you devise the most diverse diet that is likely to control FODMAP-related symptoms.

It's important to note that during the study described above, people on the low-FODMAP diet significantly reduced their intake of important nutrients. And eliminating FODMAPs doesn't just rob you of flavorful and healthy food choices; a low-FODMAP diet reduces the variety of healthful bacteria in the gut.

Because the low-FODMAP diet can be tricky to navigate, it's best to work closely with a registered dietitian who is very familiar with the diet and can help you work through the three phases of the program. A summary of FODMAP dietary guidelines is available in the patient care section of the American Gastroenterological Association website (www.gastro.org).

A colonoscopy or flexible sigmoidoscopy (procedures that involve viewing the inside of the colon with a scope inserted through the anus) can reveal tumors or inflammatory bowel disease (see "What else could it be, if it isn't IBS?" on page 20). You can have sigmoidoscopy in the doctor's office with no sedation. The doctor examines the rectum and sigmoid colon using a scope and may also take a tissue sample. To rule out colon cancer, or to screen for it in someone over age 50, the doctor may order a colonoscopy, a more involved procedure in which a scope is used to view the full length of the colon. An alternative is a computed tomography (CT) colonography, also known as a virtual colonoscopy, although some insurance companies do not cover this test when it's used to screen for colon cancer.

Not every person with a gut problem will need every test. On the other hand, everyone ages 50 and over should be screened for colon cancer (see Table 2, page 21). Besides flexible sigmoidoscopy, colonoscopy, and CT colonography, another option for screening in people at average risk for colon cancer is to test the stool for occult (hidden) blood.

Managing IBS

Because there is no cure for IBS, treatment aims to control individual symptoms. This requires a great amount of cooperation between doctor and patient. People need to educate themselves about IBS and receive adequate information from their physicians so they can learn to manage the syndrome and regain control over their lives. Such measures can have a real impact.

Self-help

You can play an active role in managing your own condition. Begin with these measures.

Identify—and then eliminate—triggers. What we know is that something has disrupted the normal functioning of the bowel in people with IBS. The trigger could be emotional stress, for example, or it could be a dietary irritant. One place to start the search is with something you've consumed—foods, beverages, or drugs, for example. Food allergy testing has not proved to be useful in identifying triggers. Once you've pinpointed your triggers, try to eliminate them.

Eat fiber. Adding fiber to your diet may help to increase the stool's bulk and speed its movement through the digestive tract. A high-fiber diet doesn't always improve bowel symptoms, and for a few people, it may increase bloating or gas. But many clinical trials have shown that it does seem to relieve constipation and may ease abdominal pain, and sometimes it even improves diarrhea. You can increase the fiber in your diet by eating plenty of fresh fruits and vegetables. An analysis of 14 studies found that supplements containing soluble fiber, which attracts water and forms a gel that slows down digestion, reduces IBS symptoms, while insoluble fiber (such as bran) is of little value for many people with IBS. Soluble fiber supplements containing psyllium or methylcellulose are available in many products found in supermarkets or drugstores and can be highly effective. For some people, this may be all that's needed to reduce symptoms.

When introducing fiber to your diet, do so gradually. Too much, too fast can cause excessive gas, cramping, and bloating. Drink lots of water or other liquids to avoid constipation.

Try heat. For people who experience IBS intermittently, a home heating pad can be a simple and inexpensive way of soothing abdominal pain. Heat can help relax cramping muscles. Similarly, drinking a warm, noncaffeinated tea such as chamomile may help reduce discomfort.

Psychotherapy

Because IBS symptoms are sometimes related to anxiety or stress, cognitive behavioral therapy (CBT) to reframe negative thoughts into more positive, productive ways of thinking can improve some people's symptoms and quality of life. Although other types of talk therapy can lessen symptoms of anxiety and depression in people with IBS, studies have shown that CBT provides the greatest improvement in overall daily functioning. One study found that people with moderate to severe IBS who participated in CBT enjoyed considerable improvements in symptom severity after six months, compared with people who did not have the therapy.

Medications for IBS

If you have symptoms that are troublesome enough to stop you from participating in normal activities, talk with your doctor about drug therapy. While medications can't cure IBS, they may ease the symptoms. Depending on your particular symptoms, your doctor might select from the following classes of drugs.

Antispasmodics. These medications, including enteric-coated peppermint oil, dicyclomine (Bentyl), or hyoscyamine (Levsin), may provide some temporary relief of mild abdominal pain by reducing bowel spasms. People who often experience cramps after eating may reduce symptoms if they take one of these drugs before meals.

Antibiotics. A substantial percentage of people with IBS who don't have constipation have an overgrowth of bacteria in their small intestines. Research shows treatment with antibiotics to eliminate this overgrowth may help improve symptoms. Based on three large trials, the antibiotic rifaximin (Xifaxan) was approved by the FDA in 2015 for the treatment of IBS with diarrhea.

Antidepressants. Tricyclic antidepressants are sometimes prescribed to treat IBS pain. Doctors suspect that the benefit of these drugs is unrelated to their antidepressant effects. People who have pain-predominant IBS may take tricyclics such as amitriptyline (Elavil, Endep) and desipramine (Norpramin) at doses lower than those used for depression. Because these antidepressants can cause constipation, they should be used only by people who have diarrhea- or pain-related IBS symptoms.

Selective serotonin reuptake inhibitors (SSRIs), such as fluoxetine (Prozac), do not control pain as effectively as the tricyclics, but they have become more popular for treatment of IBS because they tend to cause fewer side effects. SSRIs help to relieve the anxiety and depression that is sometimes associated with moderate or severe IBS, so they may be a good

Understanding food intolerance and food allergies

Food intolerance and allergies often produce similar symptoms (and symptoms similar to those of IBS), but they're not the same. A food allergy is an immune system reaction to a substance that is not normally dangerous to the body. Food intolerance, on the other hand, is not an allergic response and doesn't involve the immune system, but rather some other issue, such as inadequate amounts of an enzyme to digest a particular type of food. Two common types of food that cause intolerance are dairy products, which contain a sugar called lactose, and certain grain products, which contain a protein called gluten.

Lactose intolerance

Lactose intolerance is difficulty digesting lactose, the primary sugar found in milk. It's been estimated that up to 70% of the world's people are lactose intolerant, although the problem is minor for most. The difficulty occurs when a person's body does not produce enough of the enzyme lactase, which breaks milk sugar down into simpler forms that can be absorbed into the bloodstream. Typically, symptoms of lactose intolerance appear as soon as 30 minutes after you consume milk products. You may develop gas, diarrhea, bloating, cramps, or nausea.

The best way to avoid the symptoms of lactose intolerance is to avoid milk products. But if you don't wish to make that concession, you can take a lactase enzyme preparation, such as Lactaid, when eating foods containing lactose. There are also now dairy products (including milk, yogurt, and ice cream) that already have been treated with the enzyme. Other people who don't have as severe a problem may find that they can eat some milk products as long as they consume them with other foods. Yogurt (with live cultures) and aged cheeses may not cause as many problems as other milk products, probably because some of the lactose breaks down during fermentation. Despite widespread claims that consuming raw (unpasteurized) milk aids lactose intolerance, a 2014 study demonstrated that the practice does not reduce symptoms or aid lactose absorption. Many stores sell alternatives to milk products made from soy, rice, almonds, or other substitutes.

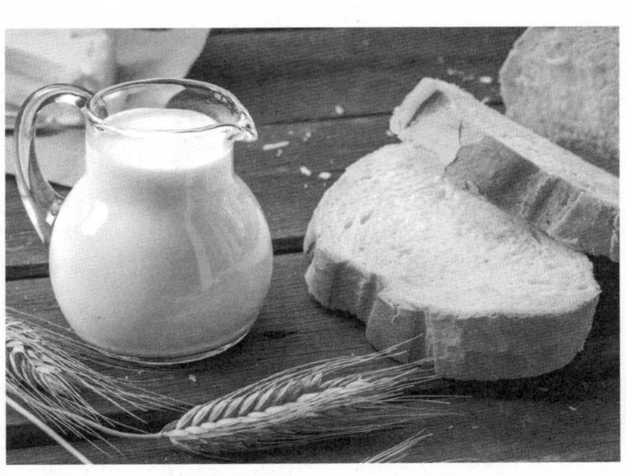

Many people are unable to digest the lactose in milk. The gluten in wheat can also cause problems, even in people without celiac disease.

Gluten intolerance

Another food intolerance centers on difficulties in digesting the grain protein called gluten. This protein is found in foods containing wheat, rye, and barley. In sensitive people, ingesting gluten can cause bloating, gas, abdominal distension, and diarrhea. Gluten intolerance is distinct from celiac disease, which is an immunological reaction to gluten. But in both cases, avoiding gluten-containing foods will eliminate the problem.

In some people, a seeming intolerance to gluten may actually be caused by a reaction to certain carbohydrates that are also found in gluten-containing grains (see "Should you stop eating FODMAPs?" on page 25). For example, in a 2017 study, people who reported gluten sensitivity were challenged with muesli bars containing either gluten, the carbohydrate fructan, or a placebo. Without knowing the contents, they reported the most IBS symptoms when consuming the fructan-containing bars, with no difference in symptoms between gluten and placebo ingestion.

treatment option for people with IBS who also have those psychiatric diagnoses.

Antidiarrheals. Loperamide (Imodium) and diphenoxylate with atropine (Lomotil) are generally recommended for people whose main symptom is diarrhea. Loperamide, available over the counter, reduces the secretion of fluid by the intestine. Diphenoxylate, which is related to codeine and available by prescription only, helps to slow down intestinal contractions. Because diphenoxylate can be habit-forming, atropine is added to the formula to cause unpleasant side effects if you take it in larger-than-prescribed quantities.

Laxatives. Many clinicians think that some laxatives, including the polyethylene glycol preparation (Miralax) used for colon cleansing prior to colonoscopy, are safe and effective for IBS when used judiciously. However, laxatives with stimulant properties like bisacodyl (Dulcolax, Correctol) or senna (Ex-Lax) may cause cramping.

Other medications. Linaclotide (Linzess) is used to treat constipation in people with IBS. It relieves intestinal pain and helps stool move more quickly through the colon. The most common side effects include diarrhea, flatulence, and abdominal pain and distension.

Lubiprostone (Amitiza) is a prescription medication first approved to treat adults who have persistent severe constipation without an identifiable cause and who have not responded to traditional therapies. The FDA later extended approval of this drug to treat women ages 18 and older who have constipation-predominant IBS. Known as a chloride-channel agonist, it enhances production of chloride-rich fluid in the gut. The most common side effects of lubiprostone are nausea, diarrhea, abdominal pain, and headache.

Eluxadoline (Viberzi) is a prescription medication approved in 2015 to treat adults who have IBS with diarrhea. The medication acts on various opioid receptors in the gut, and it lessens bowel contractions to relieve both diarrhea and abdominal pain. The most common side effects are constipation and nausea, but few people discontinue the drug because of these problems. The most serious side effect is pancreatitis, a sometimes-fatal inflammation of the pancreas. This risk is greater if you have had your gallbladder removed, and in 2017 the FDA warned that people without a gallbladder should not take eluxadoline.

Research is also focusing on the gut-brain connection, which appears to play a role in IBS. Among the medications being investigated are serotonin-like drugs known as 5-hydroxytryptamine-receptor agonists. The first of these to be approved for diarrhea-predominant IBS was alosetron (Lotronex), which works on the serotonin type 3 receptor. However, Lotronex was temporarily taken off the market in 2000 because of colitis and severe constipation that resulted in 44 hospitalizations and five deaths. Lotronex is now available for women with severe IBS with diarrhea and bowel urgency, but only under a tightly controlled prescribing program.

Probiotics and prebiotics. Probiotics are live microorganisms used to benefit health. Prebiotics are nonliving substances intended to promote the growth of the beneficial microorganisms by serving as food for them. The promise of probiotic and prebiotic treatments for gastrointestinal and other ailments is growing as scientists understand more about the important role that the microbes living in and on the human body have on health (see "A living colony in your gut—that's a good thing," page 4, and "A new treatment for IBS?" at left).

People with gastrointestinal disorders, including IBS, are prime targets for the many popular yogurts, supplements, fruit juices, and other products marketed as having probiotic or prebiotic ingredients. In a 2015 analysis combining data from 15 controlled trials on probiotics, researchers found that the products reduced pain and other IBS symptoms for some people, with those consuming probiotics being twice as likely to improve in their overall symptoms compared with those taking a placebo. There was not enough evidence to identify specific strains of bacteria as most beneficial.

Since there is currently no way to predict which people with IBS may benefit from probiotics, or how much, some gastroenterologists suggest regular consumption of fermented foods, such as sauerkraut and yogurt, along with a trial of probiotic supplements

A new treatment for IBS?

A disordered balance of bacteria within the small intestine is thought to be a factor in creating IBS symptoms. Transferring stool from a healthy donor (known medically as fecal microbiota transplantation) is a recognized approach to treating people infected with the bacterium *Clostridium difficile,* which can cause severe diarrhea. It has also been suggested as a means to restore balance and relieve IBS symptoms. However, the first preliminary randomized controlled trials of this approach, reported in 2018, had mixed results. Swallowing fecal microbiota capsules did not improve symptoms more than placebo in people with diarrhea-prominent IBS, but fecal microbiota delivered by a tube through the nose into the small intestine did improve symptoms in people with bloating-prominent IBS. More studies are needed before this approach can be recommended.

that contain *Lactobacillus* or *Bifidobacterium* to see how symptoms respond.

Although safe for most healthy people, probiotics are live microorganisms that pose concerns for people with certain medical conditions, including people at risk of invasive infections, people with an abnormal gastrointestinal mucosa barrier, those with central venous catheters, people who are immunocompromised, children with short gut syndrome, and all critically ill patients in intensive care units.

As for prebiotics, the rationale for their use in IBS seems sound, but the quality of the scientific studies is too poor to provide meaningful evidence for their use. Certain prebiotics contain fructan, one of the FODMAPs that worsen IBS symptoms in some people.

Integrative therapy for IBS

People with IBS frequently turn to health care approaches developed outside of traditional Western medicine, usually used together with conventional medicine, an approach called complementary or integrative medicine. These therapeutic approaches range from herbal remedies to meditation. Research shows that some people experience improvement through any of several stress reduction techniques taught by psychologists or other medical professionals. However, little evidence of benefit exists for most of the herbal therapies or other supplements.

Relaxation response training and meditation. Simple to do and easy to learn, these techniques help reduce nervous system activity and relax muscles. Therapies that induce a similar response include progressive muscle relaxation and guided imagery.

Yoga. Yoga, the ancient Indian discipline that seeks to bring body and mind into balance, has proved valuable to some IBS sufferers. In a 2016 analysis combining results from several small studies, people who practiced yoga had fewer and less severe IBS symptoms and lower anxiety than those undergoing conventional treatment. Yoga, like meditation, can serve as a form of self-relaxation.

Hypnosis. Increasing evidence suggests that this mind-relaxation technique calms the autonomic nervous system and might contribute to improvement in symptoms. Gut-directed hypnotherapy is intended to bring you to a very relaxed state and then provide suggestions and visualizations to minimize your symptoms. In one 2016 study, gut-directed hypnotherapy relieved IBS symptoms as well as a low-FODMAP diet.

Biofeedback. Biofeedback is a mind-body technique in which participants use a machine to see and learn to control their body's responses to stimuli such as pain. Some people who periodically lose control of their bowels, for example, have been able to improve their control using biofeedback techniques. In one study, women with difficult-to-control IBS had less anxiety and depression and fewer digestive symptoms after three sessions of biofeedback.

Acupuncture. This system of applying small needles to prescribed points on the body has been used for treatment of IBS symptoms. In a 2017 study, more than 40% of participants reported improvement in their symptoms. However, there was no significant difference between the sham and real acupuncture groups, implying a substantial placebo effect.

Herbal remedies. A growing number of people with IBS are turning to herbal remedies, including St. John's wort, fish oils, flaxseed oil, aloe vera juice, chamomile tea, and a variety of Chinese herbs. However, there are few high-quality studies that support the safety and effectiveness of such remedies. One possible exception is peppermint oil. When investigators analyzed data from nine placebo-controlled studies, they found that peppermint oil capsules or softgels significantly improved abdominal pain and overall IBS symptoms. The most common side effect was heartburn, but this was not a problem in a 2016 trial using triple-coated peppermint oil (IBgard) designed for sustained release in the small intestine. Peppermint oil may work by blocking calcium channels, thereby relaxing smooth muscles in the walls of the intestine.

Some evidence has emerged for the use of Chinese herbal preparations, but once again, the quality of the studies is not sufficient to support use of these therapies. Because most herbal preparations do not undergo rigorous scientific study, be alert to the possibility of unexpected side effects or drug interactions if you take an herbal remedy.

The stress connection

Have you ever had a "gut-wrenching" experience? Do certain people or situations make you "nauseous" (metaphorically speaking)? Have you ever felt "butterflies" in your stomach? We use these expressions to describe emotional reactions because the digestive tract is sensitive to emotion. Anger, anxiety, sadness, elation: all of these emotions and many others can trigger symptoms in the gut (see "Gut reactions," page 32). As noted already, stress is also connected in many cases with gastrointestinal ailments such as dyspepsia and irritable bowel syndrome (IBS).

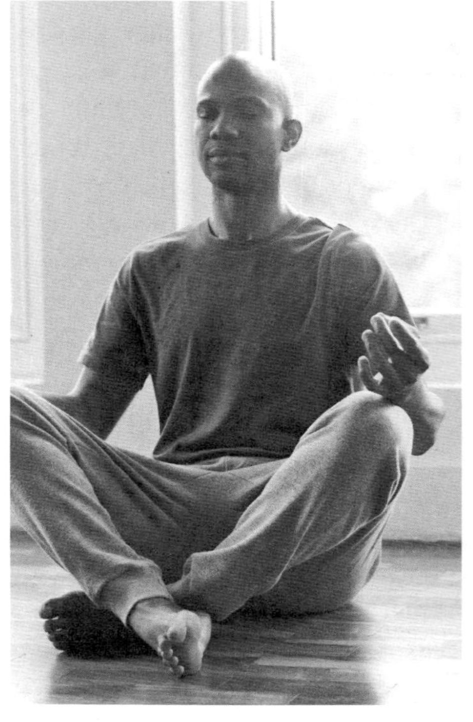

Relaxation techniques engage the body's parasympathetic nervous system, sometimes called the "rest and digest" system.

The brain has a direct effect on the stomach: even the thought of eating can release the stomach's juices before food gets there. This connection goes both ways. A troubled intestine can send signals to the brain, just as a troubled brain can send signals to the gut. Therefore, a person's distressed gut can be as much the cause as the product of anxiety, stress, or depression. That's because the brain and the gastrointestinal system are intimately connected—so intimately that they should be viewed as one system, rather than two.

This is especially true in cases when the gut is acting up and there's no obvious physical or infectious cause. For such functional gastrointestinal (GI) disorders, trying to heal a distressed gut without considering the impact of stress and emotion is like trying to improve an employee's poor job performance without considering his or her manager and work environment.

The second brain

To appreciate the impact of stress on the gut, it helps to understand the similarities and connections between the brain and the digestive system. The gut is controlled by the enteric nervous system (ENS), a complex system of about 100 million nerves that oversees every aspect of digestion. The ENS is heavily influenced by the central nervous system (CNS), with which it communicates through pathways of nerves. The "second brain," as the ENS is sometimes called, arises from the same tissues as the CNS during fetal development. It has many structural and chemical counterparts in the cranial brain, including sensory and motor neurons as well as glial cells, which support and protect the neurons.

And the ENS uses many of the same neurotransmitters, or chemical messengers, as the CNS.

The ENS is embedded in the gut wall and participates in a rich dialogue with the brain during the entire journey of food through the 30-foot-long digestive tract. The ENS cells in the lining of the gut communicate with the brain by way of the autonomic nervous system, the part of the nervous system that controls the body's vital functions. As part of that system, one set of nerves (the sympathetic nerves, which govern the "fight or flight" response) carry impulses from the gut to the spinal cord and then to the base of the brain. Another set of nerves (the parasympathetic nerves, which counter the sympathetic system and are sometimes called "rest and digest" nerves) transmit signals to the base of the brain via the vagus nerve from the upper gut or through the sacral nerves from the colon. The transmission is bidirectional; the gut and brain use their shared neurotransmitters, including acetylcholine and serotonin, to transmit information back and forth by way of these two nerve systems.

This two-way communication system between the gut and the brain explains why you stop eating when you're full (sensory neurons in your gut let your brain know that your stomach is distended), or conversely, why anxiety over this morning's exam has ruined your appetite for breakfast (the stress activated your fight-or-flight response, inhibiting gastrointestinal secretion and reducing blood flow to the gut).

Stress and the functional GI disorders

Given how closely the gut and brain interact, it might seem obvious that the pair often influence each other. Some people feel nauseated before giving a presentation; others feel intestinal pain during times of stress. In any case, emotional and psychosocial factors play a role in functional GI disorders.

That doesn't mean, however, that functional GI illnesses are imaginary, or "all in your head." Psychology combines with physical factors to cause pain and other bowel symptoms. In particular, childhood trauma such as physical or sexual abuse makes functional GI disorders more likely to occur in adulthood (see "Antidepressants to treat the body as well as the mind," page 34). Psychosocial factors influence the actual physiology of the gut, as well as the modulation of symptoms. In other words, stress (or depression or other psychological factors) can affect movement and contractions of the gastrointestinal tract, as well as sensations perceived to come from the gut. There is also emerging evidence that psychosocial factors may alter the types of bacteria that live in your gut, cause inflammation, or make you more susceptible to infection.

In addition, research suggests that some people with functional GI disorders perceive pain more acutely than other people do because their brains do not properly regulate pain signals from the digestive tract. In other words, stress can make the existing pain seem even worse.

These observations suggest that at least some people with functional GI conditions might find relief with therapy to reduce stress or treat anxiety or depression. And sure enough, one review of 32 studies showed that people treated with psychologically based approaches had greater improvement in their symptoms compared with people who received conventional medical treatment.

Treating the whole body

Stress-related symptoms in the gastrointestinal tract vary greatly from one person to the next, and treatment can vary as well. For example, one person with gastroesophageal reflux disease might have an occasional, mild burning sensation in the chest, while another experiences excruciating discomfort night after night. As the severity of symptoms varies, so should the therapies, medications, self-help strategies, or even surgeries used to relieve them.

Many people have mild symptoms that respond quickly to changes in diet or medications. If your symptoms do not improve, your clinician may ask you more questions about your medical history and perform some diagnostic tests to rule out a physical abnormality, infection, or cancer. For some people, symptoms improve as soon as a serious diagnosis, like cancer, has been ruled out (another example of how emotional stress affects the gut). Your doctor may also recommend symptom-specific medications. But sometimes these treatments are not enough. As symptoms become more severe, so does the likelihood that you are experiencing some sort of psychological distress.

Often, people with moderate to severe symptoms, particularly those whose symptoms arise from stressful circumstances, stand to benefit from psychological treatments such as cognitive behavioral therapy, relaxation techniques, and hypnosis. Some people are reluctant to accept the role of psychosocial factors in their illness. But it's important to know that emotions cause genuine chemical and physical responses in the body that can result in pain and discomfort. Behavioral therapy and stress reduction treatments do not directly reduce pain or improve symptoms in the way that drugs do. Rather, the goal is to reduce anxiety, encourage healthy behaviors, and help people cope with the pain and discomfort of their condition.

Integrative therapy for functional GI disorders shifts the focus away from pinpointing a specific cause for symptoms to engaging patients in activities and therapies that can help in managing symptoms and increasing quality of life. This may include the use of medications, dietary changes, and various techniques to reduce stress.

Gut reactions

Early researchers relied on some remarkable yet basic observations to learn how the digestive tract responds to emotions. In 1833, William Beaumont, a U.S. Army surgeon, was given an inside view when Alexis St. Martin, a French Canadian traveler, was accidentally shot in the stomach. The wound left a gastric fistula (opening to the skin) that allowed Beaumont not only to observe the pumping, to-and-fro motion of the stomach but also to see what happened when his patient expressed different emotions.

In his journals, Beaumont wrote that when St. Martin showed fear, anger, or impatience, his stomach mucosa grew pale and produced less gastric juice. Studies have since found that powerful emotions can evoke both increases and decreases in stomach secretions.

In another experiment, conducted in the 1950s, a student agreed to let medical researcher Thomas Almy view his sigmoid colon, the section of the lower colon near the rectum, through a sigmoidoscope. During the exam, someone else present mentioned cancer of the colon, and the startled student leapt to the conclusion that this was his diagnosis. The researchers watched the lining of his colon blush and contract rapidly, only to relax and regain its normal color when the student was reassured that he did not have cancer.

Cognitive behavioral therapy

Cognitive behavioral therapy, or CBT, involves working with a therapist to reframe negative ways of thinking and behaviors that affect your symptoms and quality of life. The goal is to change counterproductive thoughts and actions and learn new coping skills. This may be accomplished through a number of techniques, including changing negative thought patterns, learning stress management and relaxation techniques, modeling healthy behaviors, and role playing. CBT can reduce the stress of dealing with a functional GI disorder so that the disorder is no longer the focal point of your life. As stress decreases, symptoms often improve, and in turn stress and anxiety improve even further. In fact, in a study of people with IBS, 77% of those who underwent seven weeks of CBT reported symptom relief lasting for six months, compared with improvement in 21% of people receiving usual treatment. Helping people change their negative perceptions of IBS was particularly important in achieving benefits.

Many mental health professionals practice CBT, including psychologists, psychiatrists, social workers, and psychiatric nurses. Most cognitive behavioral therapists are not specifically trained in treating IBS or other functional GI disorders unless they are associated with a clinic that specializes in treating these conditions. More likely, you will be taught more general techniques that you can apply to your specific situation. To find a trained cognitive behavioral therapist, consult your doctor or health plan, or visit the website of the Academy of Cognitive Therapy at www.academyofct.org. Make sure your therapist has a license to practice in your state.

Is stress causing your symptoms?

When assessing whether your gastrointestinal symptoms—such as heartburn, abdominal cramps, or loose stools—are related to stress, watch for these other common symptoms of stress and report them to your clinician as well.

Physical symptoms

- Stiff or tense muscles, especially in the neck and shoulders
- Headaches
- Sleep problems
- Shakiness or tremors
- Recent loss of interest in sex
- Weight loss or gain
- Restlessness

Behavioral symptoms

- Procrastination
- Difficulty completing work assignments
- Changes in the amount of alcohol or food you consume
- Taking up smoking, or smoking more than usual
- Grinding teeth
- Rumination (frequent talking or brooding about stressful situations)

Emotional symptoms

- Crying
- Overwhelming sense of tension or pressure
- Trouble relaxing
- Increased desire to be with or withdraw from others
- Nervousness
- Quick temper
- Depression
- Poor concentration
- Trouble remembering things
- Loss of sense of humor
- Indecisiveness

Relaxation therapy

Relaxation therapy helps people to be less tense when confronting pain or stress. Therapists use a variety of methods, including progressive muscle relaxation, mental imaging, music, and even aromas, to induce a natural state of relaxation. During and after relaxation therapy, thoughts begin to flow slowly and naturally, muscle tension diminishes, and breathing slows and becomes deeper and more regular. This allows the parasympathetic ("rest and digest") nervous system to take over. The result? The body can relax and proceed with digestion.

For people with functional or stress-related GI disorders, relaxation therapy can help manage the stress associated with physical discomfort. One small study, for example, found that people with IBS who learned to elicit the relaxation response—an approach developed by Dr. Herbert Benson, founder of the Benson-Henry Institute for Mind Body Medicine—enjoyed significant short- and long-term reductions in pain, bloating, diarrhea, and flatulence. In another study that involved the Benson-Henry Institute as well as the Gastrointestinal Unit at Massachusetts General Hospital, people with IBS and inflammatory bowel disease had fewer symptoms after taking a course that combined learning and practicing the relaxation response with the development of cognitive skills to cope with stress and their gastrointestinal symptoms. In a demonstration of the powerful effect of the mind on the body, they were found to have changed the expression (activity level) of genes involved in inflammation and the digestive system's response to stress.

Many relaxation programs (including the one used in the Massachusetts General Hospital study) incorporate mindfulness, a practice of learning to observe what's going on in the present moment without judging it or thinking about the past or future. In IBS, this can mean noting your present gastrointestinal symptoms without thinking back to the worst symptoms you ever had or worrying about what may happen next. In one study of 70 people with IBS, after a mindfulness-based stress reduction program, 70% of the participants had a significant drop in their IBS symptoms, along with reduced anxiety and a higher quality of life.

There are many relaxation techniques, including yoga, meditation, hypnosis, and biofeedback. The Harvard Special Health Report *Stress Management* explains many techniques for tamping down stress levels. (To order, go to www.health.harvard.edu or call 877-649-9457, toll-free.) Many types of health care professionals, including psychologists and behavioral therapists, teach relaxation skills. Ask your doctor for a referral.

Antidepressants to treat the body as well as the mind

A small minority of people have severe functional GI symptoms that can be debilitating, significantly affecting their day-to-day lives. It's important for these people to be screened for anxiety and depression. People with severe symptoms have a high frequency of psychological diagnoses, such as anxiety, depression, or a history of loss, abuse, or trauma. In some studies, high rates of past sexual and physical abuse have been found in people with functional GI disorders—as high as 56% among people with severe symptoms. And among people referred to gastrointestinal clinics—usually those with more severe symptoms—functional bowel disorders often started after a time of extreme stress.

If either anxiety or depression appears to be a factor in a functional GI disorder, specific treatment for anxiety or depression, including referral to a mental health professional, may be needed. Moreover, people with severe gastrointestinal symptoms, especially those with chronic pain, may benefit from treatment with antidepressants even if they are not depressed. Although these medications are most often prescribed to help alleviate depression and anxiety, they also alter the function of nerves and, in lower doses, act to relieve pain. One analysis of people with IBS found that those treated with antidepressants showed an improvement in abdominal pain scores compared with placebo. Antidepressants also improve overall well-being in people with functional GI disorders. And they can help gut motility (the rhythmic contractions of the gut).

Three groups of antidepressant medications can be used to treat functional GI disorders: tricyclic antidepressants, selective serotonin reuptake inhibitors, and serotonin-norepinephrine reuptake inhibitors.

Tricyclic antidepressants. This class of drugs includes amitriptyline (Elavil), desipramine (Norpramin), and nortriptyline (Pamelor). At full doses, these medications have considerable side effects. However, when prescribed to treat pain, they are used at lower doses than those used for depression. Pain is, in part, a matter of perception; the brain may perceive gastrointestinal pain to be more or less severe based on how well it regulates signals coming from the digestive tract (see Figure 10, page 49). Tricyclics can turn down the level of pain perceived by the brain by acting on the neurotransmitters (dopamine, serotonin, norepinephrine, and acetylcholine) that are carrying pain impulses between the gut and the brain. They can also act directly on the gut, reducing the sensitivity of the gut to painful stimuli. In addition, they affect motility (constipation is a common side effect, so they are helpful for individuals with diarrhea), and they help alleviate symptoms of depression.

Selective serotonin reuptake inhibitors (SSRIs). These include citalopram (Celexa), paroxetine (Paxil), sertraline (Zoloft), and fluoxetine (Prozac). SSRIs are less effective than tricyclics for pain, but they have fewer side effects. They are a good treatment option for people with functional GI disorders who also have depression or anxiety.

Serotonin-norepinephrine reuptake inhibitors (SNRIs). Duloxetine (Cymbalta) is one example of this class of antidepressants. These drugs act on serotonin and norepinephrine, without the side effects of full-dose tricyclics. Although there are only a few preliminary studies on the effectiveness of SNRIs in fighting functional GI disorders, they are being used by some doctors in this context.

Constipation

Constipation is characterized by infrequent bowel movements or the difficult passage of dry, hard stool. It's one of the most common gastrointestinal complaints in the United States, responsible for more than 2.5 million visits to health care providers each year. The problem is more common in women than men, and more common among older people.

How constipation happens

The hard, dry stool that characterizes constipation in some people develops when the colon absorbs too much water from the stool. This may happen because the muscle contractions of the colon are too slow, so the stool moves along sluggishly. Or it can occur when the anal sphincter fails to relax when it should, causing an excessive amount of stool to be stored in the rectum. Constipation can also occur when you deliberately hold back bowel movements. If you routinely override the urge to defecate by consciously constricting the external sphincter muscles that surround the anus, your reflex to defecate may be blunted, and accumulated stool may harden as a result, becoming even more difficult to pass.

Eventually, the colon tries to move the stool by squeezing down to push it along. This causes an uncomfortable pressure and cramping. If the stool is not eliminated, more hard stool accumulates. When the stool finally passes, it can cause extreme discomfort.

Do you have functional constipation?

The Rome IV criteria for a diagnosis of functional constipation state that people must have experienced two or more of the following symptoms for the past three months, and that symptoms must have begun at least six months before diagnosis:

- ✔ straining during at least one out of four bowel movements
- ✔ having lumpy or hard stools during at least one out of four bowel movements
- ✔ having a sensation of incomplete evacuation in at least one out of four bowel movements
- ✔ having a sensation that your rectum or anus is blocked during at least one out of four bowel movements
- ✔ resorting to manual maneuvers such as using a finger to help remove feces or apply pressure to support the pelvic floor during at least one out of four bowel movements
- ✔ fewer than three defecations a week.

The diagnosis also requires these two conditions:

- ✔ no loose stools without the use of a laxative
- ✔ no diagnosis of opioid-induced constipation
- ✔ no diagnosis of irritable bowel syndrome (no prominent pain or bloating).

Causes of constipation

Many factors can dispose a person to constipation. Some can easily be prevented by changing habits and lifestyle (although the role of lifestyle factors may not be as important as once thought). Often, the cause has to do with physiological problems or diseases. Following are the more common causes of constipation:

Lack of exercise. People who exercise regularly generally don't develop constipation. Basically, the colon responds to activity. Good muscle tone in general is important for regular bowel movements. The abdominal wall muscles and the diaphragm all play a crucial role in the process of defecation. If these muscles are weak, they're not going to be able to do the job as well. But exercise is not a cure-all. Increasing exercise to improve constipation may be more effective in older people, who tend to be more sedentary, than in younger people.

Opioids. The digestive tract has receptors for opioids, and constipation can occur (or worsen) when people take opioid pain medications. Opioid-induced constipation occurs in roughly 94% of cancer patients taking opioids for pain and 41% of people taking opioids for chronic noncancer pain.

Other medications. Constipation is a side effect of many prescription and over-the-counter drugs. These include antacids that contain aluminum, antispasmodics, antidepressants, tranquilizers and sedatives, bismuth salts, iron supplements, diuretics, anticholinergics, calcium-channel blockers, and anticonvulsants.

Irritable bowel syndrome (IBS). Some people who suffer from IBS have sluggish bowel movements, straining during bowel movements, and abdominal discomfort. Constipation may be the predominant symptom, or it may alternate with diarrhea. Cramping, gas, and bloating are also common.

Abuse of laxatives. Laxatives are sometimes used inappropriately, for example, by people suffering from anorexia nervosa or bulimia. But for people with long-term constipation, the extended use of laxatives may be a reasonable solution. In the past, long-term use of some laxatives was thought to damage nerve cells in the colon and interfere with the colon's innate ability to contract. However, newer formulations of laxatives have made this outcome rare (see "Over-the-counter oral laxatives," page 37).

Changes in life or routine. Traveling can give some people problems because it disrupts normal diet and daily routines. Aging often affects regularity by reducing intestinal activity and muscle tone. Pregnancy may cause women to become constipated because of hormonal changes or because the enlarged uterus pushes on the intestine.

Ignoring the urge. If you have to go, go. If you hold in a bowel movement, for whatever reason, you may be inviting a bout of constipation. People who repeatedly ignore the urge to move their bowels may eventually stop feeling the urge.

Not enough fiber and fluids in the diet. A diet too low in fiber and fluids and too high in fats can contribute to constipation. Fiber absorbs water and causes stools to be larger, softer, and easier to pass. Increasing fiber intake helps cure constipation in many people, but those with more severe constipation sometimes find that increasing fiber makes their constipation worse and leads to gassiness and discomfort.

Other causes. Diseases that can cause constipation include neurological disorders, such as Parkinson's disease, spinal cord injury, stroke, or multiple sclerosis; metabolic and endocrine disorders, such as hypothyroidism, diabetes, or chronic kidney disease; bowel cancer; and diverticulitis (see "Diverticular disease," page 20). A number of systemic conditions, like scleroderma, can also cause constipation. In addition, intestinal obstructions, caused by scar tissue (adhesions) from past surgery or strictures of the colon or rectum, can compress, squeeze, or narrow the intestine and rectum, causing constipation.

Frequency of bowel movements: What's normal?

What is regularity? The idea that you've got to move your bowels each day to be healthy is a myth, not a medical fact. In fact, as far back as 1909, the British physiologist Sir Arthur Hurst said it wasn't unusual to find healthy people who had a bowel movement three times a day or once every three days. Today, that's still the range that's considered "normal." But many perfectly healthy people don't even fall within this broad range. In 1813, the British physician William Heberden described a patient who "never went but once a month." He also described a patient who relieved himself 12 times a day. Both patients seemed perfectly content with their bowel habits.

The truth is that everyone experiences variations in how often they move their bowels. Menstruation, vigorous physical exercise, diet, travel, and stress can all cause temporary changes in bowel habits. More important than the number of bowel movements is the consistency of the stools as they pass, the effort needed to expel them, any associated symptoms, and changes in frequency.

Functional constipation

Occasionally, people experience constipation that persists for many months, years, or decades, even though no physical abnormality of the bowel can be detected. This condition, called functional constipation, is more common in women and with increasing age.

Diagnosing constipation

Diagnosing constipation might sound simple, but in order to determine what's causing the problem—particularly if it persists—your doctor will need to ask questions about your health and symptoms and perform a physical exam. He or she will ask what medications

Over-the-counter oral laxatives

Depending on the type, oral laxatives work in a variety of ways to ease the passage of stool through the rectum. For more detail on many of these products, see the Appendix.

Bulk-forming agents. These fiber-based products take a day or so to work but are very effective and safe to take indefinitely on a daily basis. Take them with plenty of liquid. They include

- bran (in food and supplements)
- calcium polycarbophil (FiberCon and others)
- methylcellulose (Citrucel and others)
- psyllium (Metamucil and others).

Stool softeners merge with stool and soften its consistency.

- Docusate (Colace, Surfak, others) is generally safe for long-term use.
- Mineral oil should be pharmaceutical-grade (look for USP or laxative instructions on the label). However, it should not be used daily because it reduces absorption of fat-soluble vitamins. Also, it can cause lung damage if it is accidentally inhaled.

Osmotic agents are salts or carbohydrates that promote secretion of water into the colon. They are reasonably safe, even with prolonged use. They include

- lactulose (Constulose, Cholac, others)
- polyethylene glycol (Miralax)—shown to be helpful in children with functional constipation and in adults with constipation.

Saline laxatives attract and retain water in the intestine, increasing pressure and release of stool. They include

- magnesium hydroxide (milk of magnesia)
- magnesium sulfate (Epsom salts).

Stimulant laxatives act directly on the intestinal lining to elicit more vigorous contractions of the colon and secretion of water and some electrolytes. They're best used for occasional constipation. They include

- bisacodyl (Correctol, Dulcolax, Ex-Lax Ultra, others)
- casanthranol (included in Dialose Plus, Peri-Colace)
- cascara (included in Naturalax)
- castor oil (Purge)
- senna (Ex-Lax, Fletcher's Castoria, Senokot, others).

A unique side effect of some stimulant laxatives, those in the class known as anthraquinones (casanthranol, cascara, senna), is pseudomelanosis coli—a darkening of the lining of the colon seen on colonoscopy. However, pseudomelanosis coli is not associated with altered colon function and appears to be a harmless consequence of long-term stimulant laxative use.

you are taking, in case one of them could be contributing to the problem.

The physical exam may involve a visual and hands-on examination of your abdomen for any masses or tenderness. Your doctor may also perform a digital rectal exam (insertion of a gloved finger into the rectum) to feel for polyps or other abnormalities and to assess the strength of the anal sphincter muscle. He or she may perform one or more tests to help determine if there's a blockage in the colon or an underlying condition such as hypothyroidism.

Evaluating constipation may require special tests, although current guidelines from the American Gastroenterological Association recommend that your physician see how you respond to therapy before deciding if they are necessary. Tests may include any of these (in the order in which they are usually done):

Colonic transit study. For this test, on one or more days you swallow a capsule at breakfast that contains tiny indigestible rings that can be seen on an abdominal x-ray. By counting the rings remaining in your colon after five days, your doctor can determine whether stool is passing through your colon at a normal speed.

Anorectal manometry. To prepare for this test, you may be asked to use an enema or take laxatives to empty your colon. Then, while you lie on your side, the practitioner inserts a slim flexible tube (catheter) with a balloon attached into your rectum. The catheter is used to measure the pressure of anal contractions and to record the sensations you feel as you squeeze, relax, and push. The test detects abnormal muscle or nerve function that may be contributing to your symptoms, including a lack of coordination between the push to expel feces and the opening of the anal canal to let it out.

Balloon expulsion test. Usually performed in conjunction with anorectal manometry, this test involves inserting a balloon into your rectum and then filling the balloon with fluid until it reaches the size of a stool. You sit on a toilet-like seat and try to expel the balloon. The test measures the time and effort this process takes. If the test is normal, it lessens concern about the significance of any anatomical problems or lack of muscle coordination found in the anorectal manometry test.

Defecography. To prepare for this test, you use an enema—sometimes more than one—to empty your colon. Then the radiologist inserts barium contrast medium (which is visible on x-ray) into your rectum and takes x-rays while you sit on a special toilet-like seat and then attempt to pass the material. By seeing the position and movement of your rectum and anus, the radiologist can identify obstructions, prolapse (protrusion of the rectum through the anus), bulging of the rectum through weakened muscle layers, or spasms of the anal sphincter.

Treating constipation

People suffering from constipation should start by boosting fiber and fluid intake and increasing physical exercise. Drinking more water or other nonalcoholic, noncaffeinated beverages may reduce the need for the colon to rehydrate stools and is, in any case, harmless. Prune juice, warm juices, teas, and hot lemonade are often recommended. Exercise, which is widely believed to promote regularity (although few studies have investigated this), has many other health benefits as well.

Bowel training is another option. To retrain your bowel, you attempt to defecate at a regular time each day, when bowel movements are most likely to occur (such as first thing in the morning, following exercise, or after a meal). The idea is to repeat the routine until the body adopts the bowel movement as part of its daily rhythm. Although bowel training is harmless and helps some people, it has not been widely tested.

Dietary fiber and supplements

For many people, adding fiber to the diet is a highly effective way to prevent or treat constipation. The Food and Nutrition Board of the Institute of Medicine recommends 38 grams of fiber per day for men and 25 grams per day for women ages 50 and younger; for men and women over 50, they recommend 30 and 21 grams per day, respectively. Most Americans ingest much less fiber than these recommended amounts.

Good sources of fiber include whole-grain foods, brans, fruits, and vegetables. Depending on the brand, a bowl of high-fiber bran cereal delivers approximately 4 to 12 grams of fiber. Fiber supplements and other products containing psyllium seed or methylcellulose are also quite effective. Follow the directions on the label carefully as you mix the powder with a large glass of water or juice. Drinking plenty of liquid is most important when using these products. Some people find that drinking a second glass of water or juice afterwards boosts effectiveness. If liquid formulations are difficult for you to ingest, psyllium and methylcellulose are also available in capsule and tablet forms.

Laxatives

For thousands of years, people have been using various substances to help ease the passage of stool through the bowel (see "Over-the-counter oral laxatives," page 37). Under most circumstances, laxatives should be used only when dietary and behavioral measures fail. Most of the time, oral laxatives will be sufficient, but sometimes other approaches are needed.

Suppositories. Suppositories have been used to aid evacuation since the days of ancient Egypt, Greece, and Rome. Glycerin suppositories are made of about 70% glycerin, sometimes with sodium stearate (a fatty acid) added. After insertion, a glycerin suppository stimulates the reflex to defecate, in part because of its lubricating action. Suppositories with bisacodyl (Dulcolax) are more potent and usually produce a bowel movement within 20 minutes.

Enemas. The simple tap water enema distends the rectum, mimicking its natural distension by the stool, and prompts the reflex that opens the sphincters to empty the rectum. While it isn't ideal to rely on artificial stimulation to kick off evacuation, occasional use can be safe and effective. Sodium phosphate (Fleet) enemas are available in single-dose plastic containers. These salts draw fluid into the bowel, prompting intestinal contraction. Oil-containing enemas are sometimes prescribed as softeners for feces that have become hardened within the rectum. They are generally recommended for short-term use only. Avoid soapsuds enemas, which can irritate the lining of the colon.

Prescription medications

In recent years several additional drugs, known as pro-secretory drugs, have become available to treat constipation. Using different mechanisms, these agents cause additional fluid to be secreted into the intestine, maintaining stool at a consistency that is easier to pass. These drugs include the following:

- **Lubiprostone (Amitiza),** a chloride-channel agonist, is approved for functional constipation, IBS with constipation, and opioid-induced constipation. Lubiprostone may be a good option for people who are not helped by standard treatments. However, side effects such as nausea and diarrhea are frequent, and its long-term effects are unknown.
- **Linaclotide (Linzess),** a guanylate cyclase 2c agonist, is for chronic functional constipation and IBS with constipation. Diarrhea, sometimes severe, is the most common side effect.
- **Plecanatide (Trulance),** which is virtually identical to a naturally occurring peptide in the gastrointestinal system (uroguanylin), is approved for chronic functional constipation and for IBS with constipation. Diarrhea, sometimes severe, is the most common side effect.

For constipation in people taking opioids to treat chronic noncancer pain, there are now three oral medications that block opioids from binding to receptors in the gut—methylnaltrexone (Relistor), naldemedine (Symproic), and naloxegol (Movantik). An injectable form of methylnaltrexone had previously been approved for seriously ill patients receiving opioids for pain relief. Serious side effects from these medications may include symptoms of opioid withdrawal, severe abdominal pain and diarrhea, and perforation of the stomach or abdominal wall. The most common side effects are abdominal pain, diarrhea, nausea, and flatulence. Talk to your doctor about all your medications and supplements before starting any drugs to treat opioid-induced constipation, because certain combinations may increase side effects or reduce effectiveness. These drugs should not be continued after you stop taking opioid painkillers. They have not been approved for use in patients with active cancer, but may be used in patients being treated for pain related to past cancer or cancer treatment.

Biofeedback

Biofeedback can be helpful for severe constipation that results from an inability to relax the anorectal muscles and adequately straighten the angle of the rectum enough to pass stool effectively. With this method, you can be trained to relax the pelvic floor muscles during straining and coordinate this action with abdominal wall muscle contractions to enable stool to pass. About two-thirds of people with anorectal dysfunction report improvement.

Probiotics and prebiotics

A variety of probiotics and prebiotics (see page 28) have been tested for treatment of constipation, with varying results. One analysis of 14 studies found that probiotics (particularly *Bifidobacterium lactis*) sped up stool transit and frequency. However, high-quality studies establishing the efficacy of specific probiotic microbes at specific dosages are lacking. Studies have not shown prebiotics to help more than placebo in relieving constipation, perhaps because it takes time to build up a colony of microflora in the gut.

Surgery

Surgical intervention as a means of treating severe constipation is considered in a limited number of people with very severe constipation caused by a lack of colonic motility that has not responded to other treatments. The operation most commonly performed involves removing the colon and connecting the small intestine directly to the rectum. But at least half of those undergoing the procedure have had to endure additional surgery because of leaking at the junction of the small intestine and rectum, obstructions of the small intestine, or other complications.

Alternative approaches

A variety of alternative approaches are available. Solid scientific evidence is limited, but some people find flaxseed or sesame seed useful. In one study, people who used perineal self-acupressure just before defecating—pressing on the area between the anus and vaginal opening in women and between the anus and scrotum in men—reported improvements. Others have reported success using abdominal massage.

Diarrhea

Almost everyone has had a bout of "the runs" from time to time as the result of eating tainted food or drinking unclean water. Diarrhea is the body's response to something that upsets the intestines; it's the body's way of clearing out whatever is causing the upset. In most cases, the problem will resolve on its own, and you won't need to call a doctor. However, cases that don't clear up in a few days require a physician's care.

As noted earlier, diarrhea can accompany a number of gastrointestinal disorders, such as irritable bowel syndrome or ulcerative colitis. However, it may also occur on its own, intermittently or constantly.

- Diarrhea is described as acute when it lasts less than four weeks, as in viral gastroenteritis.
- It is considered chronic when it lasts four weeks or longer.
- When diarrhea occurs in more than a quarter of stools and lasts at least three months without an identifiable cause, the diarrhea is said to be functional.

Do you have functional diarrhea?

According to the Rome IV criteria, for a diagnosis of functional diarrhea, a person must have experienced the following for the past three months, with symptoms starting at least six months before diagnosis:

✔ loose (mushy) or watery stools without pain, occurring in at least one-quarter of stools.

In addition, the problem must have no identifiable cause.

While functional diarrhea has no known cause, it is important to investigate possible causes before concluding that the diarrhea is functional.

Causes of diarrhea

Normal defecation depends on the small intestine, colon, rectum, and anal sphincter working normally. The small intestine usually handles about 8 liters (roughly 8 quarts) of fluid from the diet every day and pushes about 1 liter (approximately 1 quart) of that to the colon. (The rest is absorbed into the body before it reaches the colon.) The colon absorbs most of this fluid and moves the compacted residue, which contains a few ounces of water, to the rectum. The rectum can store up to 200 grams (7 ounces) of stool before defecation is triggered. However, any interference with this process can cause the colon to be overwhelmed by the fluid load, resulting in diarrhea. In fact, any disturbance in the colon that interferes with the packing, storage, or dehydrating of the stool can result in diarrhea.

Causes of acute diarrhea

Acute diarrhea may be caused by viruses, bacteria, or parasites, as well as by various foods and drugs. It can also be a symptom of other medical conditions.

Viruses. A wide variety of viruses can cause diarrhea, which is usually short-term and resolves on its own. Among them are adenovirus, rotavirus (the most common cause of diarrhea in infants), influenza, and norovirus (the most common cause in adults). Most diarrhea is not caused by viruses, although many of the most severe cases are.

Bacteria. A number of bacteria are associated with acute diarrhea. *Shigella*, *Vibrio cholerae*, *Escherichia coli*, and *Clostridium difficile* produce toxins that cause diarrhea, while *Salmonella* and *Campylobacter* invade the stomach lining and produce inflammation and diarrhea. Food poisoning is usually due to bacterial contamination of food.

Parasites. Intestinal parasites, such as *Giardia intestinalis*, *Cryptosporidium parvum*, and roundworms or tapeworms, may cause diarrhea. These parasites are often found in untreated or contaminated water. Drinking untreated water from a lake or stream while camping is a common way to pick up *Giardia* parasites, which also cause abdominal cramps, bloating, and nausea.

Immune deficiency. People suffering from diseases such as AIDS or those who are undergoing treatments that weaken the immune system and damage the lining of the intestine, such as chemotherapy, may also suffer from severe diarrhea.

Stress. Emotions are known to wreak havoc on the bowels in a number of ways. Diarrhea is a common problem in people under severe stress or emotionally upset.

Foods. Certain foods, even if perfectly fresh, can cause diarrhea in some people. Among them are fruits, beans, and coffee. For most people, unripe fruits or any type of spoiled food will cause diarrhea, as will the particular foods that a person cannot tolerate, such as milk products for those who are lactose intolerant.

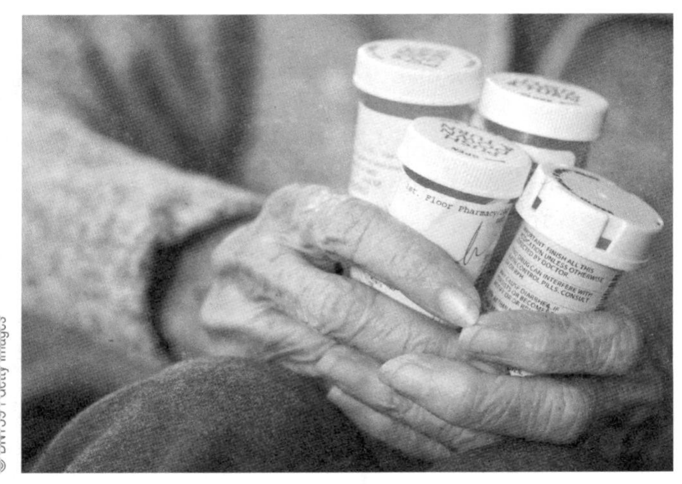

Oral antibiotics pass through the digestive tract before being absorbed into the bloodstream and can cause diarrhea by killing the "good" gut bacteria that normally keep *C. difficile* bacteria in check.

Medications. A number of prescription and over-the-counter drugs can cause diarrhea as a side effect. The most common culprits include antibiotics, antacids containing magnesium, and some blood pressure and heart medications. Because antibiotics kill some of the naturally occurring gastrointestinal bacteria, the gut becomes more vulnerable to attack by *Clostridium difficile*, a bacterium that produces toxins that can cause diarrhea. In 2005, the Centers for Disease Control and Prevention reported the emergence of a more virulent strain of *C. difficile* that causes more serious—and more often deadly—disease.

Causes of chronic diarrhea

There are numerous causes of chronic diarrhea. The condition may be an indication of irritable bowel syndrome. Chronic diarrhea may also be caused by disorders such as celiac disease or lactose intolerance that lead to the malabsorption of nutrients (see "Understanding food intolerance and food allergies," page 27). Crohn's disease and ulcerative colitis, two forms of inflammatory bowel disease, can cause diarrhea (see "What else could it be, if it isn't IBS?" on page 20).

Some forms of chronic diarrhea have nothing to do with food but are the result of excessive secretion of fluids by the intestine. These are called secretory diarrheas and may rarely be caused by tumors, sometimes in the pancreas, that release chemical messengers telling the bowel to secrete large amounts of liquid. Microscopic colitis is a more common cause of secretory diarrhea. In this case, the colon looks normal during a colonoscopy, but biopsies show intense inflammation of the colon lining.

Rarely, a person may be surreptitiously taking laxatives while seeking medical attention for chronic diarrhea, perhaps as a way of gaining attention.

In rare cases, genetic mutations can cause people to have chronic diarrhea. A report in *The New England Journal of Medicine* described 32 members of a Norwegian family who all had a gene that caused mild, chronic diarrhea. The gene appears to lead to the production of a substance that increases salt and water excretion from cells in the small intestine, causing loose stools.

When no specific cause of chronic diarrhea can be identified, the label functional diarrhea may be applied.

When to call the doctor

If your diarrhea lasts three days or more, it's time to call the doctor. However, call immediately if there is blood in the stool or if the stool looks like black tar. The same goes for diarrhea accompanied by a fever over 101° F, severe abdominal or rectal pain, and severe dehydration (symptoms include dry mouth, wrinkled skin, and lack of urination). Weight loss of more than 5 pounds is also a reason to see a doctor.

Diagnosing diarrhea

The doctor will ask questions about your symptoms and try to determine whether the diarrhea is chronic, or whether it's the result of a virus or bacterium and thus likely to be short-lived. If it's chronic, the doctor will want to probe further to establish whether the diarrhea is due to an identifiable physical problem or whether it's functional. You may be asked about your habits, including drug or alcohol use. Alcohol abuse commonly causes diarrhea, as does use of certain drugs, including cocaine.

The doctor will probably ask questions such as these:

- When did the diarrhea start?
- Have any other family members been sick?
- Have you recently traveled out of the country?
- Are you having abdominal pain? Fever? Chills?
- Is there blood in the stool?
- Is it worse when you are under stress?
- Do any specific foods make it worse?
- Do you drink coffee? Alcohol?
- What medications are you taking or have you taken recently?

If blood or pus in the stool accompanies diarrhea, or if there is fever, anemia, profound loss of appetite, or severe vomiting, it's not functional diarrhea.

For most people and for most mild episodes of diarrhea, no specific lab tests are required. But for more severe cases, or when symptoms of inflammation are present, the doctor will order stool tests to look for the presence of certain bacteria and, in some cases, parasites.

Your doctor may recommend a blood test to check for anemia, as well as testing your white blood cell count and sedimentation rate to check for signs of inflammation (see "Diagnostic tests," page 24). A sigmoidoscopy may also be performed, or a colonoscopy for people over 40. Doctors must exclude the possibility of Crohn's disease, ulcerative colitis, or other serious illness, such as colon cancer. These are often accompanied by blood in the stool, fever, or weight loss. The evaluation is likely to be more extensive if the diarrhea is chronic rather than acute and if "alarm" symptoms, such as bleeding or weight loss, are present.

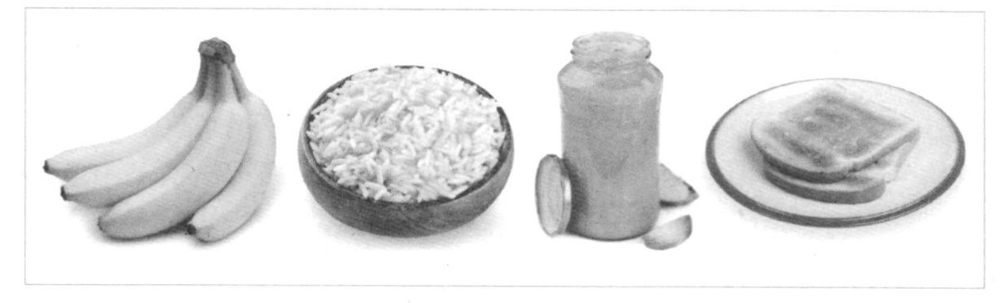

Twenty-four hours after the onset of diarrhea, you can try eating a little solid food, though a liquid diet is best. For solids, the preferred approach is a low-fiber BRAT diet, which consists of bananas, rice, applesauce, and white toast.

Treating diarrhea

Most people with acute diarrhea will recover on their own; the illness generally runs its course in a few days. In particularly severe or prolonged episodes, replacement of lost fluids and electrolytes (such as sodium and potassium) is essential to combat dehydration. Clear liquids are the first choice. For mild cases of dehydration, juices, clear broth, and safe water are recommended. Apple juice and sodas are also good choices. Citrus juices are not. Neither are alcoholic beverages.

For more severe cases, sports drinks like Gatorade can replace sugars and electrolytes, but too much may cause further diarrhea. Rehydration solutions such as Pedialyte are probably best, particularly for children with diarrhea.

Products such as kaolin and pectin (Kaopectate) give the stool a firmer consistency. Medications that work to slow the bowel include diphenoxylate with atropine (Lomotil) and paregoric, both of which are available by prescription only, as well as loperamide (Imodium), which is available over the counter. These provide quick but temporary relief by reducing muscle spasm in the digestive tract. They should be used only for a few days, however. Bismuth subsalicylate (Pepto-Bismol) also seems to work fairly well; it may temporarily turn the stool and tongue black, so don't be alarmed if that happens.

Be aware, however, that using these remedies for symptomatic relief can prolong diarrheal illness caused by infection with certain bacteria, including

Salmonella and possibly *Campylobacter*. While the medicines may make you more comfortable, they suppress the diarrhea that helps cast the offending bacteria out of your system. If you slow down the process, the bugs stay in your system longer.

After the first 24 hours, a little food is probably permissible. But it may be best to try to go without solid food as long as possible. If you are really hungry, try a BRAT diet: bananas, rice, applesauce, and white toast. The bananas bind the stool, slowing the movement a little. White rice, applesauce, and dry, white-bread toast are low in fiber and easily digested.

A wide range of probiotics and prebiotics (see page 28) have been proposed as treatment for diarrhea. The most commonly tested probiotic ingredient for diarrhea is *Lactobacillus rhamnosus GG*, available in a number of over-the-counter products (such as Culturelle Digestive Health). Some trials have shown that this probiotic shortens the duration of diarrhea. However, dose and length of treatment varied so much among the studies that no firm conclusions can be drawn. Although some probiotics may benefit people with diarrhea, the research remains too inconclusive to support specific recommendations.

Preventing diarrhea

Preventing diarrhea is largely a matter of luck and common sense. If certain foods give your intestinal tract a hard time, stay away from them. Many cases of diarrhea are caused by intestinal bugs, but if you have bouts of diarrhea not connected with bacterial infection, try to assess what foods seem to trigger it and, in particular, whether stressful situations seem connected. Keeping a diary of your food intake and diarrhea symptoms may help you make a connection with a particular food, which you can test by eliminating the possible culprit to see if symptoms improve. Take steps to reduce stress (see "The stress connection," page 30) and ask your doctor about medications that might treat functional diarrhea.

General rules for avoiding diarrhea caused by bacterial infections include washing all fruits and vegetables well and making sure they're ripe when you eat them. If you are traveling in an area where the water purity is questionable, drink and brush your teeth only with bottled water, and don't eat any uncooked fruit or vegetables. At home, cook chicken and other meats thoroughly. Clean all food preparation areas such as countertops and cutting boards with soap and warm water. Wash your hands thoroughly before and after handling food.

Be careful about eating foods left outside for long periods of time—at barbecues or picnics, for example. Bacteria can grow easily in the warm air. And don't take leftovers home from these events. Even inside, leftovers should be refrigerated quickly after the meal has been served. ■

Excessive gas

Aside from causing embarrassment, too much gas in the digestive system can result in considerable pain and discomfort—symptoms that may appear on their own or in conjunction with functional dyspepsia or irritable bowel syndrome. Sometimes you even hear and feel air and liquid swirling around inside. But there are practical steps you can take to control this problem.

Where does gas come from?

There are only two ways for gas to get into the gastrointestinal tract. Either you swallow it (aerophagia), or it's manufactured in the gut (often producing flatus).

Swallowed air

With every swallow, a little air enters the digestive tract and is transported to the stomach. To relieve pressure in the stomach and keep excess air from entering the small intestine, about 25 to 30 times each day a normal reflex causes the lower esophageal sphincter to relax and release the air in what's called a gastric belch. People with gastroesophageal reflux disease can experience frequent gastric belches, and treatment to reduce acid may help.

In contrast, a supragastric belch expels air that has just been swallowed and has not reached the stomach. The gas that erupts from the mouth usually comes from swallowed air that is forced back up. People with reflux and functional dyspepsia often swallow excess air in response to their uncomfortable gastrointestinal symptoms, leading to excess supragastric burping. Frequent supragastric belching is considered to be a learned behavior that can be changed.

Flatus

Also known as flatulence, this term describes gas that escapes from the rectum. The gas is mostly the byproduct of the fermentation of undigested food by bacteria in the colon. It contains carbon dioxide, hydrogen, and, in some people, methane. Tiny amounts of volatile chemicals produced by bacterial metabolism of residual fats and proteins are responsible for the distinctive foul odor of flatus.

Although passing gas is a natural, normal function, the resulting sounds and smells are unwelcome in social situations. The average human intestine holds 0.1 to 0.2 liters of gas, but researchers have found that in 24 hours, production of flatus averages 2 liters. This gas originates in the intestine, and its quantity and composition depend largely on the foods you eat. Studies using hydrogen breath testing have found that up to one-fifth of the complex carbohydrates eaten by average, healthy individuals is turned into gas.

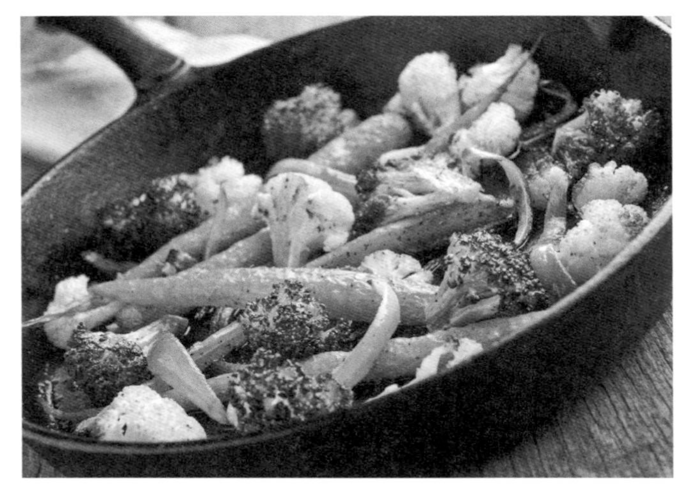

Certain foods—such as broccoli, cauliflower, Brussels sprouts, and especially beans—are notorious for causing gas. However, cooked vegetables tend to cause less gas than raw ones.

A gas primer

The air we breathe is made up mostly of nitrogen (N_2) and oxygen (O_2), the gas the human body needs to sustain life. Air that's swallowed enters the gastrointestinal tract. Another intestinal gas is carbon dioxide (CO_2), a byproduct of a chemical reaction with acid in the stomach. Hydrogen (H_2) is released in the colon when undigested carbohydrates undergo bacterial fermentation.

Bacteria in the gut produce foul-smelling gases when they ferment undigested foods that have not been absorbed in the small intestine. These foods consist mostly of carbohydrates, sugars, and fats. The carbohydrates found in high-fiber foods, such as beans, broccoli, cauliflower, and Brussels sprouts, are the worst culprits. These foods release gases such as methane (CH_4) and hydrogen sulfide (H_2S), which smells like rotten eggs. The worst odor is related to strong-smelling sulfurs, which make up just 1% of flatus.

Methane is detected in about one-third of adults. Studies show that Americans and Europeans are more likely to produce methane than Asians are, possibly because of diet. Women also produce more than men do. Genes may play a role in methane production, as the trait is passed along in families.

Additional carbon dioxide is produced in the colon as the byproduct of bacterial fermentation of unabsorbed sugars and starches. Eating beans substantially increases carbon dioxide production, as does taking sodium bicarbonate for heartburn. Thus, it doesn't make sense to use bicarbonate-containing seltzers for gas.

Foods that may cause gas

There is great variation in the foods that cause gas in different people. Some of the more common offenders are listed below.

- Apples
- Bananas
- Beans, peas, and lentils
- Broccoli
- Brussels sprouts
- Cabbage
- Carbonated beverages
- Cauliflower
- Corn
- Cucumbers
- Grapes
- Milk and other dairy products
- Nuts
- Oats and other high-fiber foods
- Onions
- Raisins
- Sorbitol
- Turnips
- Wine

Gas in the intestine

You hardly notice gas when it enters your digestive system, but once it's there, the discomfort can be intense. People who suffer the symptoms of gas pain usually have the same volume of gas as anyone else, or just a little bit more. But it affects them more because they are more sensitive. Some people with chronic gas pain have impaired intestinal peristalsis and significant reflux of gas from the small intestine into the stomach.

Although gas pain is not usually a sign of significant health problems, it is important to see a doctor if the symptoms persist or are severe because they are occasionally a sign of some more serious condition. For example, severe distension immediately following a meal, sometimes called magenblase (stomach bubble) syndrome, may be mistaken for heart pain. Splenic flexure syndrome is a painful spasm in the left upper abdomen below the rib cage, produced by localized areas of trapped gas in the colon. These conditions are treated with the same dietary modifications and medications that are used for other forms of excess gas.

Borborygmi is an onomatopoeic word that refers to sounds created by peristaltic activity. Although disconcerting to the person whose insides are grumbling, it often goes unnoticed by anyone else.

Eating habits and gas

Throughout history, certain foods have been notorious for producing gas (see "Foods that may cause gas," above). Beans are the most obvious example. Beans contain the complex carbohydrates stachyose and raffinose, which the intestine can't absorb but the bacteria in the colon love. The problem is most serious in people who have been eating a low-fiber diet and switch to a diet rich in beans and other high-fiber foods. Their digestive tracts don't have enough of the enzymes needed to digest bean sugars, which pass undigested into the colon, where the bacteria metabolize them and generate gas. If people eat beans on a regular basis, the problem usually lessens as the body begins to produce the enzymes it needs.

People who are lactose intolerant often describe distressing flatulence if they consume milk products (see "Understanding food intolerance and food allergies," page 27). Other factors, such as disturbances in motility or metabolism, also influence how often and how much flatus is passed. For instance, people with slowed intestinal motility may produce more gas simply because bacteria have more time to work their magic on complex carbohydrates. Gas production may also increase when people take antibiotics, which lead to changes in the types of bacteria in the colon, or when the acidity level in the stomach goes down, as occurs when you take a proton-pump inhibitor (see page 12).

Diagnosing air swallowing and flatus

The important thing for a doctor to consider in diagnosing a belching or flatulence problem is whether it's occurring alone or in conjunction with one or more of the various functional gastrointestinal disorders or a more serious illness. He or she should be alert to problems that may suggest a serious disease, such as weight loss or anemia. Of course, a physician may be able to determine quickly that the problem is the result of eating too many beans or swallowing too much air. In most cases, evaluating gassiness will not require extensive diagnostic testing.

To assess your gassiness, your doctor will first question you about your symptoms and dietary patterns. If upper gastrointestinal symptoms are the major problems, excessive air swallowing may be the culprit. The doctor will ask about possible lactose intolerance as well as habits such as gulping down meals, drinking carbonated beverages, sipping through a straw, chewing gum, smoking cigarettes, or chewing tobacco.

The doctor will also want to know about anxiety and psychological problems that may contribute to air swallowing and predispose people to symptoms, including gas and cramping. Likewise, he or she will want to review the medications you are taking, since some—especially drugs that are encapsulated with a sorbitol filler—can induce gas, bloating, and diarrhea.

A distended abdomen can be detected by tapping it and listening for a hollow sound. Causes of intestinal distension include obstruction of the bowel or fluid or a mass in the abdomen. But other signs usually accompany these more serious problems, and they usually can be readily confirmed by an imaging study such as a CT scan. Some can be identified with a simple abdominal x-ray. In many cases, an imaging test is not necessary. Some doctors may want to run a lactose absorption test or hydrogen breath test to check for lactose intolerance.

Bloating and distension: It's not excess gas

Your abdomen feels uncomfortably full and actually looks a bit larger than usual. Is it excess gas? Probably not. That feeling of fullness and tightness in the abdomen is called bloating, while distension is the actual increased size of the abdomen. The two conditions usually occur together—and the combination is much more bothersome than bloating alone—but it is possible to have bloating without distension.

Bloating affects 10% to 30% of the general population, with women twice as likely to experience it as men. Functional bloating is an independent diagnosis, but it is also frequently associated with other functional gastrointestinal disorders. For example, 75% of people with irritable bowel syndrome (IBS) say they have bloating; in fact, people with IBS often rank bloating as their most bothersome symptom. Bloating is also often accompanied by excessive flatulence and frequent belching.

You might think that bloating and distension come from excess gas. But more likely the discomfort is due to IBS, and the distension is the result of relaxation of the muscles of the abdomen and diaphragm (the muscle that separates the abdomen from the chest). Scientists have measured gas content and abdominal size in people who have bloating and distension and have not found that people with these symptoms have more gas than people who don't.

Abdominal wall strength or function seems to play a role. Abdominal muscles relax during meals to accommodate large volumes of food. In people who experience distension, the abdominal wall may relax to an abnormal degree, and the diaphragm may drop, causing further distension. Think of the opposite of the typical upright military posture, which requires sucking in abdominal muscles and the diaphragm to pull in the stomach and thrust out the chest. In people with distension, the diaphragm drops, abdominal muscles sag, and waist circumference grows. Excessive descent of the diaphragm may also be a factor.

There are no surefire treatments for bloating and distension, but because they often go hand in hand with IBS, they are treated the same way (see "Managing IBS," page 25).

Treating belching and air swallowing

The key to treating belching and air swallowing is to reduce the amount of air you swallow. If you chew gum or smoke, quitting should cut down on air gulping. Dentures that are too loose can also cause you to swallow air. Avoid carbonated drinks and whipped desserts, which trigger burping. Some people swear by eating certain foods, such as brown rice or barley broth. Papaya and pineapple are also said to help.

Make sure to chew foods slowly, and avoid washing food down with liquids. Try to eat smaller meals, and don't eat when you are anxious, upset, or overtired. If you have aerophagia, antidepressants and tranquilizers may help by calming the nerves or lessening anxiety, but you should use these carefully and only under a doctor's close supervision.

Taking a brisk stroll after eating, rather than taking a nap, is a good idea. It promotes gastric emptying and helps relieve the bloated feeling. When it's time to go to bed, try sleeping on your stomach or right side to aid in the escape of gas and alleviate fullness.

In cases of supragastric belching, behavioral therapy may be effective. A speech therapy program that has been developed to help people become aware of air swallowing and practice exercises to suppress the supragastric belching mechanism effectively treated the majority of patients with supragastric belching in one study.

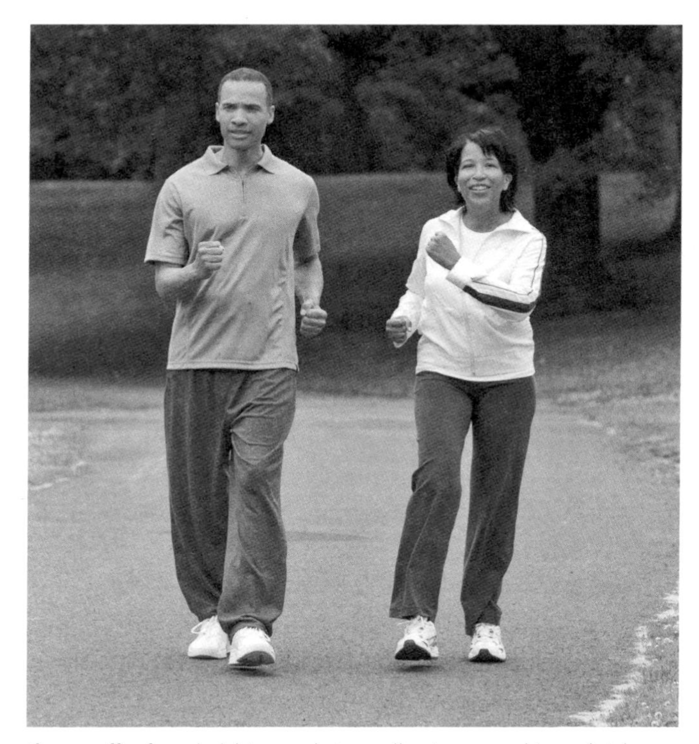

If you suffer from belching and air swallowing, try taking a brisk walk after eating. This promotes gastric emptying and helps relieve any bloated feeling you might be sensing.

Treating flatulence

The first step is to stop eating the foods that cause gas: milk, beans, fruits, and other complex carbohydrates, as well as the artificial sweetener sorbitol. But don't eliminate all fruits and vegetables, because these foods are the basis of a healthy diet. Cooked vegetables tend to cause less gas than raw vegetables. A product called Beano, which contains the enzyme alpha-galactosidase, might help metabolize difficult-to-digest complex carbohydrates when taken before meals. And preparations containing the pancreatic enzymes lipase, trypsin, and amylase, taken with meals, may reduce gassy emissions by helping to digest proteins, starches, and fats. These enzymes are sold over the counter in capsule form (a product called Super Digestive Enzymes is one example) at stores that sell nutritional supplements.

Some people find it helps to drastically reduce dietary sugars and cut back on refined starches and wheat flour. Activated charcoal, a tasteless black powder, absorbs gas and for some people reduces gassiness, particularly after a high-carbohydrate meal. Occasional use is not harmful. Additionally, Pepto-Bismol may reduce the odor of flatus.

Some people have success with anticholinergic drugs such as dicyclomine (Bentyl) and hyoscyamine (Levsin). These agents block nerves that stimulate the digestive tract. A course of the broad-spectrum antibiotic rifaximin (Xifaxan) may also help reduce flatulence, usually without side effects.

A variety of probiotics have been tried for treating flatulence, with some success, but studies so far have not been large enough or well constructed enough to support specific recommendations.

When all else fails, wearing a deodorizing and absorbing pad containing activated charcoal inside your undergarments won't stop flatulence, but it may prevent others from noticing it.

Abdominal pain disorders

Many functional gastrointestinal disorders involve pain, but some people experience constant or frequent abdominal pain that is not related to food intake (as with functional dyspepsia) or defecation (as with irritable bowel syndrome). Their pain is severe enough to interfere with the ability to function in many aspects of life, and some people undergo multiple surgical procedures in an often-futile attempt to find and correct the source of the pain. Patients often describe the pain as having a burning quality, and encompassing a larger area of the abdomen than the more localized pain from other gastrointestinal disorders.

The most recent Rome guidelines recognize two abdominal pain syndromes—centrally mediated abdominal pain syndrome and narcotic bowel syndrome.

Centrally mediated abdominal pain syndrome (CAPS). There are no imaging studies or lab tests that confirm the diagnosis of CAPS. Instead, the diagnosis is based on a careful history and physical exam. You may be surprised to be asked about trauma in your past, but there's an important reason why. Post-traumatic stress disorder (PTSD), which can occur after trauma such as a sexual assault, battlefield experience, or motor vehicle collision, has several characteristics (increased arousal, sleep disturbances, and anxiety) that can create physical pain symptoms. Many types of chronic pain, such as lower back pain and headaches in addition to abdominal pain, can stem from PTSD arising from trauma in the recent or distant past, and simultaneously addressing PTSD in general along with the specific painful trouble spot can help you gain control over your symptoms.

As you might expect from its name, the central nervous system plays a significant role in the pain of CAPS, and treatment involves taking advantage of the powerful effect of the brain on the gut in order to relieve it (see Figure 10, page 49). You may be prescribed an antidepressant at a low dose (lower than for depression; see "Antidepressants to treat the body as well as the mind," page 34), or you may try mind-body techniques such as relaxation and hypnosis to help your brain block pain messages from your abdomen. The goal of treatment is to reduce your pain as much as possible and help you return to normal activities.

Antidepressants commonly used to treat CAPS include tricyclic antidepressants and serotonin-norepinephrine reuptake inhibitors. If these fail, combinations of various drugs may be used—including atypical antipsychotics such as quetiapine (Seroquel) or aripiprazole (Abilify, Aristada), antianxiety drugs such as mirtazapine (Remeron) or buspirone (Buspar), and delta ligand agents such as pregabalin (Lyrica) or gabapentin (Neurontin).

Narcotic bowel syndrome. When opioid painkillers such as morphine and oxycodone are used for any reason, some people (an estimated 6%) have a paradoxical response; the narcotics sensitize their nerves and make pain worse. In fact, people with CAPS should not take opioids. The abdominal pain

Do you have centrally mediated abdominal pain syndrome?

The Rome IV criteria specify that centrally mediated abdominal pain syndrome must include one or more of the following for the past three months, with symptoms beginning at least six months before diagnosis:

- ✔ continuous or nearly continuous abdominal pain
- ✔ no or only occasional relationship of pain with physiological events (such as eating, defecating, or menses)
- ✔ pain limits some aspect of daily functioning
- ✔ pain is not feigned
- ✔ pain is not explained by another structural or functional gastrointestinal disorder or other medical condition (such as a gynecological problem).

Figure 10: Closing the pain gate

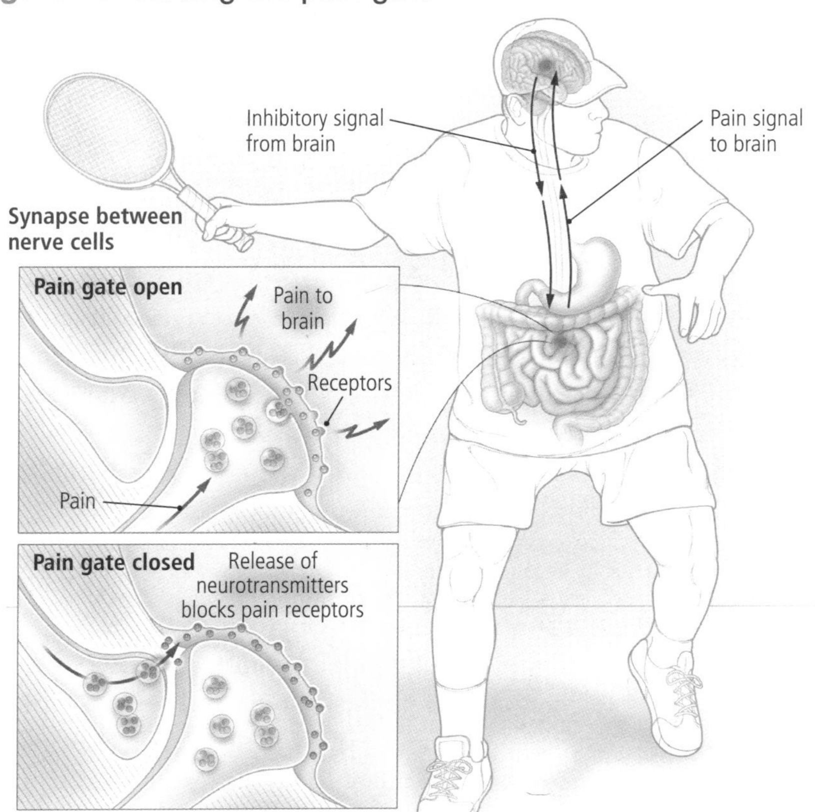

Have you ever noticed that you feel pain less when you're doing something that requires all your attention? That's because pain is not a one-way street of pain signals traveling from your gut (or elsewhere in your body) to the brain. The brain also sends messages back to the rest of the body that help modulate the sensation of pain.

Experts call this the "gate control" theory. In the case of intestinal pain, receptors (known as afferent receptors) pick up a pain signal and route it toward the brain. But certain centers in the spinal cord ("pain gates") may either allow the signal to proceed to the brain or "close the gate" and block the signal. The latter process is sometimes called "downregulation" of the pain signal. Your brain does this naturally when you are doing something that requires deep concentration, such as playing a sport intensely. Antidepressant medications can also help close the gate by blocking or inhibiting the pain signal to the brain.

never goes away and may worsen the longer they take opioids or the higher the dose they use. Hour by hour, it may seem as if the drugs are helping; as each dose of the painkiller wears off, the pain may markedly worsen and seem to improve with the next dose. But over months of use there is a progression of the frequency, duration, and intensity of pain. It can be difficult for patients, and even their physicians, to distinguish between pain that results from the narcotics and the underlying pain that is being treated. This opioid-related abdominal pain syndrome—known as narcotic bowel syndrome—may come on gradually in people who use opioids for nonabdominal pain as well.

Treatment involves the slow but steady substitution of alternative drugs to counter pain, anxiety, and depression until the opioids are completely out of your system. In a small study, detoxification led to a reduction in pain by at least 30% in about half of the patients. Those able to stay off opioids for three months afterward had a 75% reduction in abdominal pain compared with pretreatment levels.

The prevention of narcotic bowel syndrome involves avoiding the use of opioid painkillers when possible, and when necessary taking them at the lowest dose and for the shortest period of time possible. Despite the potential for adverse effects such as constipation and increased pain in people with functional gastrointestinal disorders (as well as addiction), opioids are prescribed more frequently for them than for patients with structural gastrointestinal problems. If you are offered a prescription for an opioid painkiller for your gastrointestinal symptoms, ask about the possibility of narcotic bowel syndrome. ■

Appendix: Medications for gastrointestinal disorders

These are the most common drugs used to treat various gastrointestinal disorders (including functional disorders). Pregnant or nursing women should not take these drugs, except on the specific advice of a physician.

Antacids (for acid reflux)

ACTIVE INGREDIENTS	BRAND NAME	USE	SIDE EFFECTS	COMMENTS
alumina, aluminum carbonate, aluminum hydroxide	Amphojel, Gaviscon, Maalox, Mylanta	Relieve heartburn and functional dyspepsia pain. Promote ulcer healing by neutralizing stomach acid.	Constipation, diarrhea. Excessive and prolonged doses may cause bone pain, discomfort, appetite loss, mood changes, muscle weakness.	Side effects more likely in people with kidney disease. Aluminum-containing antacids not advised for elderly people with bone disease or Alzheimer's disease. Do not use within three to four hours of taking tetracycline-type antibiotics.
calcium carbonate	Alka-Mints, Caltrate, Rolaids, Tums		Constipation. Excessive and prolonged doses may cause upset stomach, vomiting, stomach pain, belching, constipation, dry mouth, increased urination, loss of appetite, metallic taste.	Chalky taste. Side effects more likely in people with kidney disease.
magnesia, magnesium carbonate, magnesium hydroxide, magnesium trisilicate	Gaviscon, Gelusil, Maalox, Mylanta, Phillips' Milk of Magnesia		Excessive and prolonged doses may cause difficult or painful urination, dizziness, irregular heartbeat, loss of appetite, mood changes, muscle weakness.	Chalky taste. Side effects more likely in people with kidney disease. Do not use within three to four hours of taking tetracycline-type antibiotics.
sodium bicarbonate	Alka-Seltzer, baking soda		Abdominal fullness, belching. Excessive and prolonged doses may cause additional side effects.	Not advisable for people on low-sodium diets. Side effects more likely in people with kidney disease.

Anticholinergics/antispasmodics (for intestinal pain)

GENERIC NAME	BRAND NAME	USE	SIDE EFFECTS	COMMENTS
atropine with hyoscyamine, phenobarbital, and scopolamine	Donnatal*	Relieve cramps and spasms.	Dry mouth, difficulty urinating or urinary retention, blurred vision, rapid heartbeat, increased pressure inside the eye, headache, nervousness, drowsiness. Antispasmodics that contain phenobarbital may cause sedation, drowsiness, or, rarely, agitation.	Do not use if you have glaucoma. Consult your doctor if you take other medications, because these drugs block or boost the actions of many other medications. Phenobarbital may decrease the effect of anticoagulants and may be habit-forming.
dicyclomine	Bentyl*			
hyoscyamine	Levsin*			

Antidiarrheal agents (for diarrhea)

GENERIC NAME	BRAND NAME	USE	SIDE EFFECTS	COMMENTS
alosetron	Lotronex*	Reduces cramping, abdominal pain, urgency, and diarrhea caused by IBS.	Constipation. In rare cases, may cause diarrhea and intestinal bleeding.	Available only under a tightly controlled program. Only proven effective in women.
diphenoxylate and atropine	Logen,* Lomotil*	Stops diarrhea by slowing down intestinal movement.	Abdominal discomfort, constipation. Less frequently, may cause blurred vision, urinary discomfort, dry mouth or skin, rapid heartbeat, restlessness, or warm, flushed skin.	Drink plenty of fluids. May be habit-forming. Do not use with alcohol or other depressants.
eluxadoline	Viberzi*	For IBS with diarrhea, acts on opioid receptors in the digestive tract to slow intestinal movement and lessen abdominal pain.	Nausea, constipation, and abdominal pain. Serious side effects include pancreatitis and spasm of the sphincter that controls the flow of bile and pancreatic juice into the small intestine.	Do not use if you have had your gallbladder removed, have liver or pancreas problems, or have had a bowel obstruction.

** Available by prescription only.*

Antidiarrheal agents (for diarrhea) *continued*

GENERIC NAME	BRAND NAME	USE	SIDE EFFECTS	COMMENTS
loperamide	Imodium, Imodium A-D	Reduces secretion of fluid by the intestine.	Abdominal discomfort, constipation. Less frequently, may cause drowsiness, dizziness, dry mouth, nausea, vomiting, rash.	Drink plenty of fluids. Use with caution if you have liver disease.

H2 blockers (for acid reflux)

GENERIC NAME	BRAND NAME	USE	SIDE EFFECTS	COMMENTS
cimetidine	Tagamet	Relieve heartburn and functional dyspepsia pain and promote ulcer healing by decreasing stomach acid. May be used long-term following a course of PPIs.	Rarely, may cause diarrhea, constipation, dizziness, anxiety, depression, drowsiness, sleeplessness, headache, irregular heartbeat, sweating, itching, redness of skin, fever, confusion in ill or elderly people.	May interfere with the absorption of anticoagulants, antidepressants, and hypertension medications.
famotidine	Pepcid			No serious drug interactions known.
nizatidine	Axid			
ranitidine	Zantac			May interact with anticoagulants.

Laxatives (for constipation)

GENERIC NAME	BRAND NAME	USE	SIDE EFFECTS	COMMENTS
bisacodyl	Correctol, Dulcolax, Fleet, others	Increases the motility of the bowel.	Stomach cramps, upset stomach, diarrhea, stomach and intestinal irritation, fainting, irritation or burning in the rectum (from suppositories).	May cause a blackening of the lining of the colon seen on colonoscopy (pseudomelanosis coli), which appears to be harmless.
castor oil	Purge	Causes fluid to accumulate in the small intestine.	Diarrhea, upset stomach, vomiting, irritation, cramping.	
docusate	Colace, Surfak	Softens stool by merging with feces and softening consistency.	Stomach or intestinal cramps, stomach upset, throat irritation.	Generally considered safe for long-term use.
lactulose	Cholac, Constulose, others	Synthetic sugar softens stool by pulling water into the intestine.	Diarrhea, gas, nausea.	Also used to draw ammonia from blood in people with liver disease.
linaclotide	Linzess*	Relieves constipation-dominated IBS.	Diarrhea, flatulence, abdominal pain and distension.	
lubiprostone	Amitiza*	Increases the amount of fluid secreted into the bowel, allowing stool to pass more easily.	Nausea, diarrhea, bloating, stomach pain, gas, vomiting, headache. Rarely, chest discomfort and difficulty inhaling after taking a dose.	FDA-approved for chronic constipation in both men and women, but only in women for IBS with constipation. Not for use in children.
mineral oil	various	Softens stool by merging with feces and softening consistency.	May cause deficiencies of fat-soluble vitamins if used regularly. Can cause lung damage if inhaled.	Choose a pharmaceutical-grade product; look for USP or laxative instructions on the label.
plecanatide	Trulance*	Stimulates fluid secretion in the intestine to treat chronic constipation, IBS with constipation, and opioid-induced constipation.	Diarrhea, occasionally serious.	Do not use if you have gastrointestinal obstruction. Not for use in children.
polyethylene glycol	Miralax	Softens stool and increases the number of bowel movements by flushing the intestine.	Upset stomach, bloating, cramping, gas.	
senna	Ex-Lax, Fletcher's Castoria, Senokot, others	Increases motility of the bowel.	Diarrhea, upset stomach, vomiting, irritation, cramping.	May cause a blackening of the lining of the colon seen on colonoscopy (pseudomelanosis coli), which appears to be harmless.

* *Available by prescription only.*

Opioid-receptor blockers (opioid-induced constipation)				
GENERIC NAME	BRAND NAME	USE	SIDE EFFECTS	COMMENTS
methylnaltrexone	Relistor*	Relieve constipation in people taking opioids to treat severe chronic noncancer pain.	Abdominal pain, diarrhea, nausea, gas, vomiting, headache. Abdominal pain and diarrhea may be severe. Opioid withdrawal. Other serious side effects may include perforation of stomach or abdominal wall.	May interact with a variety of prescription drugs, including antivirals, certain antibiotics, and heart medications. Consuming grapefruit or grapefruit juice can raise blood levels. Review all medications and supplements you take with doctor before using. Do not use if you have had a bowel obstruction. Do not continue use after stopping opioid painkiller. Not for use during pregnancy.
naldemedine	Symproic*			
naloxegol	Movantik*			

Prokinetic agent (for stomach discomfort)				
GENERIC NAME	BRAND NAME	USE	SIDE EFFECTS	COMMENTS
metoclopramide	Reglan*	Enhances gastric emptying.	Diarrhea. Less frequently, may cause restlessness, drowsiness, muscle tremor, spasms, breast discharge. Potentially irreversible involuntary movement of limbs may occur with longer (more than 12 weeks) or higher-dose treatment.	Increases the effects of alcohol and other depressants. Use with caution if you have type 1 diabetes or Parkinson's disease.

Proton-pump inhibitors (PPIs; for acid reflux)				
GENERIC NAME	BRAND NAME	USE	SIDE EFFECTS	COMMENTS
dexlansoprazole	Dexilant*	First-line treatment for reflux esophagitis. Promote ulcer healing by suppressing secretion of stomach acid.	Rarely, may cause constipation, chest pain, headache, gas, rash, drowsiness.	Increase the risk of diarrhea associated with *C. difficile* infection. Long-term use may increase the risk of vitamin B_{12} deficiency, hip fracture, and possibly other complications. May increase risk of bacterial infection in people with liver disease. May prolong the effect of other prescription drugs. Rabeprazole, pantoprazole, and esomeprazole are available as intravenous formulations. People taking the antiplatelet agent clopidogrel (Plavix) should avoid omeprazole and esomeprazole.
esomeprazole	Nexium			
lansoprazole	Prevacid			
omeprazole	Prilosec, Zegerid			
pantoprazole	Protonix*			
rabeprazole	Aciphex*			

Selective serotonin reuptake inhibitors (SSRIs; for a variety of functional disorders)				
GENERIC NAME	BRAND NAME	USE	SIDE EFFECTS	COMMENTS
citalopram	Celexa*	Relieve chronic abdominal pain. Speed transit in the gut, a benefit in people with IBS with constipation.	Upset stomach, diarrhea, vomiting, stomach pain, drowsiness, excessive tiredness, tremor, excitement, nervousness, difficulty falling or staying asleep, muscle or joint pain, dry mouth, excessive sweating, changes in sex drive or ability, loss of appetite.	Limited experience in functional bowel disorders. May help reduce sensitivity to pain in some people.

** Available by prescription only.*

Selective serotonin reuptake inhibitors (SSRIs; for a variety of functional disorders) *continued*

GENERIC NAME	BRAND NAME	USE	SIDE EFFECTS	COMMENTS
fluoxetine	Prozac*	Relieve chronic abdominal pain. Speed transit in the gut, a benefit in people with IBS with constipation.	Rash, headache, dizziness, insomnia, anxiety, drowsiness, excessive sweating, nausea, diarrhea, bronchitis, weight loss, painful menstruation, sexual dysfunction, urinary tract infection, chills, muscle or joint pain, back pain.	Limited experience in functional bowel disorders. May help reduce sensitivity to pain in some people.
paroxetine	Paxil*		Pain, bodily discomfort, hypertension, sudden loss of strength, rapid heartbeat, itching, nausea, vomiting, weight gain or loss, central nervous system stimulation, depression, vertigo, cough.	
sertraline	Zoloft*		Nausea, trouble sleeping, diarrhea, dry mouth, sexual dysfunction, drowsiness, tremor, indigestion, increased sweating, increased irritability or anxiety, decreased appetite.	

Tricyclic antidepressants (used in low doses for pain relief)

GENERIC NAME	BRAND NAME	USE	SIDE EFFECTS	COMMENTS
amitriptyline	Elavil,* Endep*	Relieve chronic abdominal pain. Slow transit in the digestive tract, a benefit in people with IBS with diarrhea.	Dizziness, dry mouth, blurred vision, drowsiness, constipation, urinary retention, low blood pressure, irregular heart rhythm.	Do not use with alcohol, other antidepressants, or immediately following a heart attack. Side effects may be worse when cimetidine is used simultaneously. Use with caution if you have glaucoma.
desipramine	Norpramin*			
nortriptyline	Pamelor*			

Other agents (for a variety of gastrointestinal disorders)

GENERIC NAME	BRAND NAME	USE	SIDE EFFECTS	COMMENTS
activated charcoal	Actidose-Aqua, CharcoCaps	Relieves intestinal gas.	Black stools, abdominal pain.	Effectiveness uncertain. Do not take at exactly the same time as other medications.
alpha-galactosidase	Beano	Reduces intestinal gas by breaking down indigestible carbohydrates.	No known side effects.	Effectiveness uncertain.
bismuth subsalicylate	Pepto-Bismol	Relieves heartburn, indigestion, nausea, and diarrhea. Occasionally used with antibiotics to cure ulcers.	Dark tongue, grayish-black stools. Excessive doses may cause additional side effects.	Avoid if allergic to aspirin or other salicylates.
lactase	Lactaid	Prevents gas, abdominal bloating, and diarrhea by breaking down milk sugar into simpler forms.	No known side effects.	Effectiveness uncertain. Available as pills or prepared food products.
rifaximin	Xifaxan*	Prevents traveler's diarrhea caused by *E. coli*. Treats small intestinal bacterial overgrowth in IBS. Reduces flatulence and discomfort of bloating.	Headache, constipation, hives and itchiness.	Do not use if you have fever or blood in the stool.
simethicone	Gas Relief, Gas-X, Mylanta Gas	Relieves pain from excess gas.	No known side effects.	Effectiveness uncertain.

** Available by prescription only.*

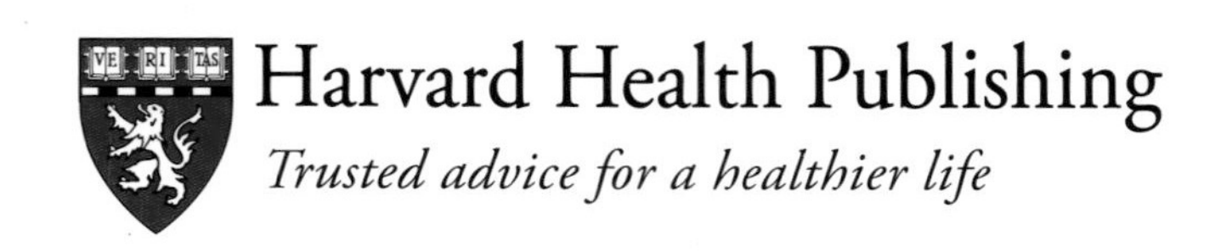

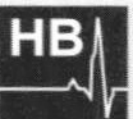

Receive *HEALTHbeat*, Harvard Health Publishing's free email newsletter

Go to: **www.health.harvard.edu** to subscribe to *HEALTHbeat*. This free weekly email newsletter brings you health tips, advice, and information on a wide range of topics.

You can also join in discussion with experts from Harvard Health Publishing and folks like you on a variety of health topics, medical news, and views by reading the Harvard Health Blog (**www.health.harvard.edu/blog**).

Order this report and other publications from Harvard Medical School

online | **www.health.harvard.edu**

phone | **877-649-9457 (toll-free)**

mail | **Belvoir Media Group**
Attn: Harvard Health Publishing
P.O. Box 5656
Norwalk, CT 06856-5656

Licensing, bulk rates, or corporate sales

email | **HHP_licensing@hms.harvard.edu**

online | **www.content.health.harvard.edu**

Other publications from Harvard Medical School

Special Health Reports *Harvard Medical School publishes in-depth reports on a wide range of health topics, including:*

Addiction
Allergies
Advance Care Planning
Alzheimer's Disease
Anxiety & Stress Disorders
Back Pain
Balance
Caregiving
Change Made Easy
Cholesterol
Cognitive Fitness
COPD
Core Workout
Depression
Diabetes
Diabetes & Diet
Energy/Fatigue
Erectile Dysfunction
Exercise
Exercise Your Joints
Eye Disease
Foot Care
Grief & Loss
Hands
Headache
Hearing Loss
Heart Disease
Heart Disease & Diet
Heart Failure
High Blood Pressure
Incontinence
Knees & Hips
Life After Cancer
Living Longer
Memory
Men's Health
Neck Pain
Nutrition
Osteoarthritis
Osteoporosis
Pain Relief
Positive Psychology
Prostate Disease
Reducing Sugar & Salt
Rheumatoid Arthritis
Sensitive Gut
Sexuality
Skin Care
Sleep
Strength Training
Stress Management
Stretching
Stroke
Tai Chi
Thyroid Disease
Vitamins & Minerals
Walking for Health
Weight Loss
Women's Health
Yoga

Periodicals *Monthly newsletters and annual publications, including:*

Harvard Health Letter
Harvard Women's Health Watch
Harvard Heart Letter
Harvard Men's Health Watch
Prostate Disease Annual

ISBN 978-1-61401-185-9

ISBN 978-1-61401-185-9
SX95000

SG0818